# The Painful Prescription

## Studies in Social Economics

TITLES PUBLISHED

STUDIES IN SOCIAL ECONOMICS

*Henry J. Aaron and William B. Schwartz*

# The Painful Prescription: Rationing Hospital Care

*A study sponsored jointly
by the Tufts University School of Medicine
and the Brookings Institution*

THE BROOKINGS INSTITUTION
*Washington, D.C.*

*Library of Congress Cataloging in Publication data:*

Aaron, Henry J.
   The painful prescription.

   (Studies in social economics)
   Includes bibliographical references and index.
   1. Hospital care—United States.   2. Hospital care—
Great Britain.   3. Hospital utilization—United States.
4. Hospital utilization—Great Britain.   5. Medical
policy—United States.   6. Medical policy—Great Britain.
I. Schwartz, William B.   II. Title.   III. Series.
[DNLM: 1. Health policy—United States.   2. Health
services needs and demand—Economics—United States.
3. Cost control.   4. Economics, Hospital—United States.
5. State medicine—Great Britain.   WX 157 A113p]
RA981.A2A5   1984      362.1′1′0973      83-45962
ISBN 0-8157-0034-2
ISBN 0-8157-0033-4 (pbk.)

9 8 7 6

THE BROOKINGS INSTITUTION is an independent organization devoted to nonpartisan research, education, and publication in economics, government, foreign policy, and the social sciences generally. Its principal purposes are to aid in the development of sound public policies and to promote public understanding of issues of national importance.

The Institution was founded on December 8, 1927, to merge the activities of the Institute for Government Research, founded in 1916, the Institute of Economics, founded in 1922, and the Robert Brookings Graduate School of Economics and Government, founded in 1924.

The Board of Trustees is responsible for the general administration of the Institution, while the immediate direction of the policies, program, and staff is vested in the President, assisted by an advisory committee of the officers and staff. The by-laws of the Institution state: "It is the function of the Trustees to make possible the conduct of scientific research, and publication, under the most favorable conditions, and to safeguard the independence of the research staff in the pursuit of their studies and in the publication of the results of such studies. It is not a part of their function to determine, control, or influence the conduct of particular investigations or the conclusions reached."

The President bears final responsibility for the decision to publish a manuscript as a Brookings book. In reaching his judgment on the competence, accuracy, and objectivity of each study, the President is advised by the director of the appropriate research program and weighs the views of a panel of expert outside readers who report to him in confidence on the quality of the work. Publication of a work signifies that it is deemed a competent treatment worthy of public consideration but does not imply endorsement of conclusions or recommendations.

The Institution maintains its position of neutrality on issues of public policy in order to safeguard the intellectual freedom of the staff. Hence interpretations or conclusions in Brookings publications should be understood to be solely those of the authors and should not be attributed to the Institution, to its trustees, officers, or other staff members, or to the organizations that support its research.

# Foreword

For three decades the cost of hospital care has been rising at a rate exceeding that of inflation or the growth of population. The principal force driving increases in inflation-adjusted hospital expenditures is the rapid growth of medical technology. Continued technological advances, together with rising incomes and the aging of the population, promise further increases in hospital costs. These trends largely account for the rise in the price of private health insurance; they also explain the growth of medicare and medicaid. Thus the rising cost of hospital care is straining both the private and the public purses.

Much of this growth has gone for dramatically effective diagnostic and therapeutic devices. But a growing share has gone for the purchase of services that produce nothing of perceptible value, or only marginal benefits, at high cost. In an effort to curb such outlays, the federal government has recently launched a program to pay hospitals on a prospective basis according to the patient's diagnosis, age, and certain other factors for services rendered under the medicare program. Several states have imposed limits of various types on the reimbursement of hospitals. But these efforts are too recent to permit a considered judgment on how effective they will be in restricting useless or low-benefit care. It is also too early to characterize fully the changes in behavior and the choices that will result from sustained and successful efforts to slow the growth of hospital spending.

To gain some insight into what will happen if budget limits are indeed sustained and successful, Henry J. Aaron and William B. Schwartz examined how the British, who spend about half as much per capita as U.S. citizens do on hospital care, have responded to tight budget limits. They use the British experience as the basis for drawing inferences about how Americans would respond should they undertake to sharply reduce growth of medical spending. After describing the British health care system, Aaron and Schwartz examine ten important medical procedures, most of which have been developed in the past two decades, and compare the ways in which they have been applied in Britain and the United States. They find that, though some forms of care are provided in Britain at the same rate as they are in the United States, the British health care system rations most hospital services in varying degrees.

The authors infer the values and perceived benefits that led to the particular pattern of sacrifices that now prevails in Britain. In the final chapter they consider how rationing would work in the United States— what form it might take, what benefits would be given up, and what American reactions might be. They note that enforcement of limits on medical spending would be much more difficult in the United States than in Britain for various reasons—political and class structure, the organization of the delivery of medical care, the prevalence of fee-for-service practice in the United States and its absence in Britain, and the deeply held presumption of most American patients that all possible care will and should be made available to them. An article based on parts of this book appeared in the *New England Journal of Medicine,* vol. 310 (January 5, 1984).

Henry J. Aaron is a senior fellow at the Brookings Institution and professor of economics at the University of Maryland. William B. Schwartz is Vannevar Bush University Professor and professor of medicine at Tufts University and senior physician at the New England Medical Center. They are grateful to Susan Eysmann, Bernice Golder, Lisa James, Alice Keck, Linda Kole, and Diane Levin, who provided research assistance; to Penelope Harpold, who checked the manuscript for accuracy; to Kathleen Elliott Yinug, who typed the manuscript; to Caroline Lalire, who edited it; and to Florence Robinson, who prepared the index. This project was carried out under grants from the Health Care Financing Administration and the National Center for Health Services Research to the Brookings Institution, and from the Robert Wood Johnson Foundation to Tufts University.

The views expressed here are the authors' alone and should not be ascribed to the University of Maryland, Tufts University, the Robert Wood Johnson Foundation, the Health Care Financing Administration, the National Center for Health Services Research, or to the trustees, officers, or other staff members of the Brookings Institution.

December 1983                                          BRUCE K. MACLAURY
Washington, D.C.                                             *President*

# Authors' Acknowledgements

We are particularly grateful to the following people who read and offered constructive comments and suggestions on the entire manuscript: Dr. William Bennett, Dr. Eugene M. Berkman, Sir Douglas A. K. Black, Peter Fox, Dr. John T. Harrington, Jeremy Hurst, Bridger Mitchell, Dr. James Mongan, Sir J. D. N. Nabarro, Joseph P. Newhouse, Dr. Gilbert S. Omenn, Joseph A. Pechman, Robert Piron, Louise B. Russell, Frank A. Sloan, Dr. William C. Waters, Professor Oliver M. Wrong.

Scores of other experts in the United States and Britain also assisted us in the preparation of this volume through correspondence, provision of documents, or comments on various sections of the book. Indeed, without the active cooperation of officials at the U.K. Department of Health and Social Security, physicians, other staff, and administrators in the National Health Service, and many other British experts this book would have been impossible to write. With apologies to those whose names we have inadvertently omitted, we wish to acknowledge the assistance of Brian Abel-Smith, Dr. Michael Alderson, Dr. Kenneth D. Bagshawe, Dr. Raphael Balcon, Professor Roger J. Berry, Gwyn Bevan, Dr. Ronald D. Bradley, A. Burchell, Graham Calder, Professor J. S. Cameron, Professor Stewart J. Cameron, Dr. P. S. Clarke, Harold Copeman, Dr. Adrian J. Crisp, Professor Derek Crowther, Dr. Thomas Deeley, R. G. Deighton, Professor Robert B. Duthie, Michael J. Fairey, Christine Farrell, T. A. Farwell, Joan Firth, Dr. E. C. Gordon-Smith, Clifford Graham, Dr. David L. Gullick, David Hand, John Harley, Alan Healey, Dr. Peter Hennesley, Colin Hetherington, Professor Walter W. Holland, Rupert P. S. Hughes, John H. James, Patrick Jenkin, Professor Ivan D. A. Johnston, Dr. Peter Jones, Richard J. Kent, Dr. Louis Kreel, William Laing, R. C. Lawson, Michael Lee, Dr. A. Fenton Lewis, Dr. T. J. McElwain, Gordon McLachlan, Dr. J. Melters, Dr. W. J. Modle, Dr. R. F. Mould, C. A. Muir, Dr. Ronald M. Oliver, Professor Michael

Peckham, John Perrin, Dr. G. Pincherle, Dr. Ray Powles, Dr. M. J. Prophet, Dr. Charles R. C. Rizza, J. A. Rowntree, William Rush, W. J. W. Sarrard, Professor James A. Scott, Dr. Walter Somerville, Dr. Edgar Sowton, Professor J. D. Swales, Dr. Mary Tate, Dr. Diana Walford, Patsy Wright Warren, Ian Wickings, Professor Alan Williams, Dr. Anthony J. Wing, Dr. R. J. Wrighton.

We wish to thank the following American experts for advice and assistance: Ernest Anderson, Dr. Henry Banks, Dr. Bengt Bjarngard, Dr. Philip Bondy, Dr. Mortimer M. Bortin, Dr. Murray F. Brennan, Dr. George P. Cannellos, Dr. Barbara Carter, Dr. Philip Cole, Dr. Modestino Criscitiello, Dr. Thomas E. Davis, Dr. Vincent T. DeVita, Jr., Dr. James P. Diamond, James A. Donahue, Dr. Joseph D. Ferrone, Dr. Robert P. Gale, Dr. Richard Gorlin, William Gouveia, Dr. William E. Hathaway, Dr. Samuel Hellman, Dr. Andrew S. Levey, Dr. Arthur S. Levine, Dr. Herbert J. Levine, Dr. Peter Levine, Dr. Nicolaos E. Madias, Dr. Hywel Madoc-Jones, Dr. Ronald A. Malt, Dr. Charles G. Moertel, Dr. Larry Nathanson, Dr. Stephen W. Papish, Dr. Robert E. Paul, Lance Piccolo, Dr. Anthony F. Piro, Dr. Charles Pross, Alice Rivlin, Dr. Richard Rudders, William Rush, Dr. Thomas P. Ryan, Dr. Deeb Salem, Dr. Robert Sarno, Joseph M. Sceppa, Dr. Lucius Sinks, Dr. Thomas P. Smith, Dr. Ezra Steiger, Dr. Edward S. Sternick, Dr. E. Donnall Thomas, Dr. Henry Wagner, Leon P. Wateska.

Many other people—physicians, staff of health teams, and others— met with us for extended discussions during our trips to Britain. Their number is so large, however, that regretfully we cannot attempt to include their names.

H.J.A.

W.B.S.

# Contents

*part one* **Introduction**

# chapter one The Promise and the Problem

The good news is that modern medicine can work miracles. The bad news is that it is very expensive and that many health expenditures do not seem to yield benefits worth their cost. Medical expenditures in the United States (in 1982 dollars) rose from $503 per capita in 1950 to $776 in 1965 (the last pre-medicare, pre-medicaid year) and to $1,365 in 1982, 10.5 percent of gross national product.[1]*

Such explosive growth reflects the enormous improvement in medical science but also arouses fear that Americans may be spending more than is desirable. For most commodities such a rise in spending would not provoke the concern that surrounds the growth in outlays on health care. The doubling of real spending on computers between 1968 and 1980, for example, is hailed as a sign of technical and scientific advance. It does not elicit fretful handwringing about spiraling computer expenditures or demands for containing computer costs.

The reason is not only that the price of computation has been dropping steadily and dramatically. After all, the price of enabling people crippled by arthritic hips to walk again has dropped from infinity (hips simply could not be replaced until the late 1960s) to about $10,000. The price of pinpointing the exact location of many deep cancers or abscesses with CT scanners or ultrasound is measured now in hundreds of dollars rather than, as previously, in the pain, cost, and risk of exploratory surgery and extended hospitalization.

The purchase of computers differs from the purchase of health care in that computer buyers pay for each additional machine they buy, whereas most patients pay very little for additional services. To be sure, patients pay increased insurance premiums or taxes to support health programs as national expenditures rise, but these increases are not

* Numbered footnotes begin on p. 139.

3

directly related to the care they receive as individuals. The cost to the patient of additional care is usually small because 90 percent of hospital costs are covered by private insurance, government programs, or payments from someone other than the patient. This insulation of the patient from the cost of care, a deliberate goal of public policy in recent decades, has led to what many feel are excessive hospital expenditures; the debate on how to limit such expenditures reflects the success of that policy.

### Efforts to Limit Hospital Expenditures

The growth of expenditures on medical care, in general, and hospital care, in particular, has led several administrations to propose limits on hospital outlays or other restrictions on the growth of medical spending. President Richard M. Nixon launched his economic stabilization program on August 15, 1971, by freezing all prices and wages for ninety days. His phase II controls, which lasted from November 1971 to April 30, 1974, contained detailed and complex limits on the allowable increase in revenue per day of hospital care, or patient day.[2]

The 1978 budget of Gerald R. Ford requested Congress to limit the rate of increase in per diem reimbursements to hospitals and in the charges made by physicians under both the medicare and medicaid programs.[3] The limit was to be 7 percent or the actual rate of increase in the preceding year, whichever was less. But the incoming administration of Jimmy Carter withdrew the Ford proposals on the ground that they would create a lower standard of care for the poor, the aged, and the disabled than for other patients—a two-class, discriminatory system.

As an alternative to the Ford budget initiatives, the Carter administration proposed a limit on the increase in total inpatient revenues of nonfederal short-term hospitals—one that would apply to all patients, not just to those covered by medicare and medicaid.[4] The life of this proposal was short. After hearings in four committees and extensive negotiations among administration officials, representatives of interest groups, and members of Congress and their staffs, the House of Representatives on November 15, 1979, rejected the Carter bill and voted instead to set up a national commission to study the problem of hospital costs.

The administration of Ronald Reagan, upon entering office in 1981, declared that it would undertake its own measures to control the increase in expenditures under the medicaid and medicare programs. Besides advocating reductions in benefits, Reagan officials declared support, in principle, for measures designed to increase competition in the delivery of care by making patients and providers more cost conscious.

On a parallel track, Congress tried to slow the rise of medical expenditures by regulations mandating that states attempt to prevent duplication of medical facilities. By 1980 all states except Louisiana required health care providers to obtain a "certificate of need" (CON) from the local health systems agencies before making a capital expenditure greater than $100,000 or $150,000. Failure to obtain a certificate of need disqualified a health care provider from reimbursement under medicaid or medicare. In principle, a certificate of need is granted only if facilities offering similar services do not exist in the same general area, or if existing facilities are operating at or above the rates set by Department of Health and Human Services (HHS) guidelines and by individual states.

Evaluation studies showed that CON programs slow the increase in numbers of beds; but the funds saved are simply moved to new services and equipment, so that there is no perceptible effect on overall hospital costs. Moreover, savings in older CON programs, in which the accumulation of experience might lead to improved results, are no greater than in new ones. Of equal concern, other research suggested that the prevention of all duplication would achieve only modest, one-time savings, which would not affect the subsequent rate of increases in cost. Because of these studies and because of an antipathy to government regulation, the Reagan administration sought in 1982 to terminate the CON programs, but Congress extended the authorization for one year.[5]

Meanwhile, state governments have been experimenting with ways to hold down medical expenditures. By 1979 eight states had introduced mandatory programs to reduce the rate of growth of hospital expenditures.[6] These programs control hospital charges, third-party payment rates, or total hospital revenue, and hospitals are forced to absorb any costs beyond their allowed level of reimbursement.

Such state controls appear to hold down the rate of growth of hospital costs by about 3 percent a year, but only after the programs have been in place for at least three years.[7] The results thus stand in sharp contrast to the ineffectuality of the certificate-of-need programs. But the critical questions concern the ability of reimbursement limits to make a real dent in hospital costs. Will the states that have adopted controls be willing to sustain them as they bite deeper into expenditures that would have been made in their absence? Does the political will to curb growth of hospital expenditures exist outside the states that have adopted controls?

Such questions are not merely academic. In 1982 Massachusetts enacted legislation limiting expenditures of all hospitals, with a sufficient reduction over a six-year period to hold the growth of hospital expenditures to 7.5 percent below the rate of inflation.[8] And in March 1983 Congress enacted legislation giving the federal government increased power to control hospital costs. The legislation mandates that a fixed sum be paid for any given diagnosis under the medicare program and places the hospital at risk if it spends more than the stated amount.

### Lessons from Britain

In contrast to the United States, Britain has drastically curtailed the real growth of medical expenditures for an extended period.* As a result, per capita hospital expenditures are now less than half as large as those in the United States, even after adjustment for salary differences. In imposing these limits, the British have encountered problems and made choices that the United States will face if it should undertake to sharply limit medical expenditures. An examination of those experiences can provide lessons from which the United States can learn.

For various reasons British patients and physicians may have responded differently to tight constraints on health expenditures from the way that their American counterparts would respond. But there are also reasons to expect similarities. A shared language has made the medical journals of each country common reading in the other. The clinical and scientific standards have been nearly identical in both countries. Under a longstanding tradition, many physicians from each country spend time in the other as students, teachers, and researchers.

The differences are important, however. Some are the result of

---

* Great Britain includes England, Wales, and Scotland; the United Kingdom includes Northern Ireland as well. In this book some data refer to England, some to England and Wales, some to England, Wales, and Scotland (that is, Great Britain), and some to the United Kingdom. To avoid confusion, we use Britain as the general term. Where precision of reference is necessary, we indicate the correct entity in the text or in a footnote.

differences in the availability of resources. Others, of course, are due to important differences between British and American society and medical practice—the organization of health care, the political system, and the relative importance of class, for example. These differences prevent us from using British experience as an exact script for the choices the United States would make if it sought to severely curb medical expenditures. But they do not invalidate the relevance of these experiences and choices for the United States.

As background to the analysis of these issues, in the next chapter we describe the British health care system for American readers.[9] To measure the practical results of budget limits, in chapters 3–5 we compare the levels at which various health care services are provided in the United States and Britain. We initially concentrated on high-technology procedures, mostly of recent vintage, because we thought that the need for such forms of care to compete with established procedures for resources highlights the effects of budget limits. But we later broadened our survey to include a number of older and more conventional forms of care.

For most procedures we use the level of services in the United States as a measure of the treatment that would result if all care expected to generate net medical benefits were provided. With some important exceptions, the norm for hospital care in the United States approximates the maxim "if it will help, do it." The system of third-party payment that dominates hospital reimbursement in the United States encourages the provision to most patients of all care that promises to yield benefits, regardless of cost. Most American patients are insulated from the financial consequences of most hospital episodes. Most American physicians gain financially from providing additional care, and medical ethics preclude only the delivery of care that will do harm, not of care that is unreasonably expensive. Hospital administrators seek facilities of high enough quality to satisfy the professional goals of their staffs. Thus care in the United States is usually close to what would be provided if cost were no object and benefit to patients were the sole concern.

In one sense, care in the United States falls short of full care. Several million Americans lack adequate insurance or personal means and therefore face obstacles to obtaining hospital care. Furthermore, not all hospitals have the space and equipment their staffs regard as necessary for the best possible care. As noted, budget limits have been imposed by some states in recent years, and in selected areas they seem to have caused or to promise significant reductions in expenditures. For these reasons and others, hospital care in the United States is rationed, in the sense that not all care expected to be beneficial is provided to all patients.

Some services in the United States may be provided in greater quantities than full care. Many physicians are reported to practice defensive medicine, minimizing the probability of malpractice suits by ordering tests and consultations that show due diligence but are not expected to yield any net medical benefits. Others are rumored to perform unneeded surgery or recommend unnecessary tests in order to boost their own incomes.

For most procedures that we have studied we do not have enough information to determine whether, or in which direction, actual service levels deviate from full service. In the few cases where we have evidence of overprovision in the United States, we compare British service levels with adjusted, rather than actual, levels of care in the United States. Except in those cases, we regard Britain as providing full care if it provides care as frequently and in the same general way as the United States does; we calculate how far short of full care British practice falls and try to determine whether the pattern of differences between Britain and the United States makes medical and social sense. Chapter 6 lays out an analytical framework for thinking about these questions and presents estimates of the degree to which differences in the provision of the procedures examined in chapters 3–5 account for the large difference between U.S. and British health expenditures.

### Preliminary Hypotheses

As we began our examination of responses to budget limits, we held certain hypotheses about the kind of trade-offs that budget limits would have forced the British to make. We anticipated that treatment for the elderly would be curtailed more than treatment for the young. We predicted that lifesaving treatments would be curtailed less than those that improve the quality of life. Because of the relative ease of deciding not to buy new equipment, as opposed to directly refusing care to a sick patient, we expected that treatments dependent on costly equipment would be reduced more than those dependent only on staff time and ordinary supplies. The special terror that cancer seems to arouse led us to speculate that its treatment would be curtailed relatively little. We expected that new treatments would be provided in relatively smaller amounts than old ones, because new treatments would have to compete with established services for available resources. We expected diagnostic procedures about which patients were likely to know little to be supplied in smaller amounts than procedures about which the public was better informed. In general, we expected the degree to which a service is curtailed to depend on the height and shape of the "social benefit" curve per dollar of expenditure. This concept is presented in chapter 6.

We found that most of our hypotheses seemed to be consistent with observed British behavior. On the other hand, we also realize that we have more plausible explanations for the observed patterns than we could test with the number of alternative medical procedures we examined. For this reason, we cannot claim to have tested in a statistically rigorous way our explanations for why the British limit different forms of care in such different degrees. Readers will have to decide whether we tell a plausible story about why the British have limited care as they have and whether people in the United States would respond similarly or differently.

We also found, however, some responses to budget limits by British patients and providers that we had not fully anticipated; and we found problems and responses that any nation will have to address in order to make budget limits work. Physicians, for example, have had to learn to say no in ways that are acceptable both to themselves and to their patients. Patients unwilling to accept the consequences of resource limits have found ways to "work the system" and to get care that they were initially denied. Communities have learned how to force hospitals to provide new services by donating equipment that would not otherwise be available. Interest groups have used the media to try to pressure the government to increase allocations for the treatment of certain diseases. In chapter 7 we describe the British responses. In chapter 8 we consider how these and similar responses would affect the operation of budget limits in the United States.

In chapters 7 and 8 we also address several other complex questions. First, should patients be permitted to buy medical care outside a system subject to budget limits? If there are no financial barriers to medical care, there are no budget limits; but if the barriers are unscalable and budget limits are severe, political opposition will probably rise sharply. What is a workable middle course that sustains both the limits and their continuing political acceptability?

Second, can clinical freedom survive in an environment of budget limits? Doctors jealously guard clinical freedom, the right of each practitioner to prescribe as he or she thinks best in each case. Included in this freedom is the right of each doctor to prescribe medication, and of each specialist (consultant, in British parlance) to admit and discharge patients, to prescribe tests, and to undertake or prescribe such surgical procedures as are thought likely to be beneficial. How can such freedom be preserved when the number of beds and operating rooms is curtailed, the capacity to do tests is limited by congestion resulting from reduced purchases of equipment, and budgets for drugs must compete with other high-priority hospital expenditures? Though faced with this issue daily, most British physicians have managed to preserve what they regard as clinical freedom. But British consultants are salaried hospital employees; American specialists are largely private businessmen who use the hospital as a place for doing business. Could American specialists develop working arrangements and attitudes that would allow them to preserve enough clinical freedom under budget limits to make the limits acceptable?

Third, what policies should be adopted toward charitable gifts? The offer of "free" medical equipment may impose unaffordable burdens on staffing and materials, or they may make services affordable that would otherwise be too costly for the limited hospital budget. What could be expected to happen in the United States?

Fourth, what legal actions would arise because of effective budget limits? Malpractice suits by patients would tend to increase if budget limits prevented doctors from providing care deemed standard for good medical practice. Doctors unable to gain access to operating rooms, hospital beds, or particular technologies that they deemed necessary for the proper care of patients or for earning an adequate income might also bring suit. How have the British grappled with this potential problem? How would Americans deal with it?

Finally, budget limits lead many patients and doctors to devise ways to cope with the restrictions. Some doctors learn how to commandeer scarce supplies; some patients learn how to secure more than their share of care by persistence or skill. Such kinds of behavior will cause budget limits to fall with uneven effect. Doctors who know they cannot care for all treatable patients face a tormenting dilemma. They can fight the limits, or they can accept them. If they fight them, political opposition will be likely to eventually destroy the budget limits. If they accept them, they must find a way to deny care to patients who would benefit from a treatment that budget limits put beyond reach and to get the patients to accept this situation. Equally important, doctors often find some way of persuading themselves that it is good medical practice to deny treatment to a patient who might benefit from it were it available. The British for the most part have solved these problems. It is not clear whether Americans would be equally successful.

To gather information for this book, we interviewed scores of British physicians, health administrators, and others expert on various aspects of the British health care system. These interviews supplied information and personal evaluations to supplement the data in official documents and scholarly publications. In the course of this book, we quote extensively from these interviews but do not attribute the quotations to specific people. All quotations are verbatim and are preserved on tape.

At the end of this book, readers should have a better understanding of what kinds of choices budget limits have forced on British health planners, doctors, and patients and of what stresses such budget limits have generated within the political system that imposed them. They should also be more aware of the range of issues the United States will confront if hospital budgets are curtailed. They should have begun to consider how American health planners, doctors, and patients might respond to binding budget controls on the health care system.

We shall not shed light on the many technical questions arising from different types of budget limits. Revenue limits per patient day, for example, encourage long hospital stays, whereas revenue limits per admission encourage the admission of cases that consume few resources. Rather, we focus on the kinds of decisions and trade-offs that will have to be made if budget limits are to work, the adjustments in behavior that will be encouraged, and the kinds of institutional change that will result from limitations on medical resources. We try to explore the value judgments that budget limits force us to apply and the coping mechanisms that they will elicit. But we are unsure how far the United States will—or should—venture in trying to cut back medical costs.

## chapter two  The British System


The famous exchange between Ernest Hemingway and F. Scott Fitzgerald, in which Fitzgerald remarked, "The rich are different from you and me," and Hemingway replied, "Yes, they have more money," applies also to the difference between the American and British health care systems. The American health care system costs much more than the British system—nearly three times as much per capita.[1]

The difference between health expenditures in Britain and those in the United States somewhat exaggerates the discrepancy between health care in the two countries. Doctors and nurses are paid more in the United States than in Britain, and the difference is even wider than that in average wages. But even if one assumes that none of the extra pay U.S. doctors and nurses receive reflects differences in quality, and if one excludes expenditures on research and administration that do not contribute directly to patient care in the short run, the United States still spends about twice as much on hospital care.[2]

Although Britain spends much less than the United States, it has, per capita, 12 percent fewer acute care hospital beds, 67 percent as many doctors, slightly more nurses, 70 percent as many admissions to acute care hospitals, and 25 percent longer hospital stays.[3] But, as will become clear in part 2, the British have much less of the equipment found in advanced U.S. hospitals. Crude indicators of health status put Britain abreast or slightly ahead of the United States. Life expectancy at birth for men was 70.2 years in Britain in 1979 and 69.9 years in the United States; British baby girls born in 1979 could expect to live 76.2 years, and their American counterparts about 1 year more. During the first year of life babies born in 1979 died at the rate of 12.9 per thousand in Britain and 13.1 per thousand in the United States.[4]

Such measures do not mean that the British health care system is better or worse than the U.S. system, because much health care affects the quality of life, not its duration. Furthermore, genetic and environmental factors have a strong effect on life expectancy. But these data do show that the large differences in per capita average medical expenditures between the two countries are not associated with large differences in life expectancy.

### Formation of the National Health Service

To an American, the most striking aspect of the creation of the National Health Service (NHS) in 1948 was the relative lack of controversy over the event. The British Medical Association vigorously opposed the change, but the Royal Colleges representing the various types of physicians overcame this resistance. The remarkable consensus on behalf of the NHS in part reflected the prior existence of a so-called national health system created in 1911 under Lloyd George. Through many employment-based funds, this system provided a limited set of mandatory benefits to workers. Though coverage was national, the system was full of holes. Some plans provided certain extra benefits for workers themselves, but there were no benefits for dependents (except maternity benefits for nonworking wives).[5]

World War II profoundly changed political and social attitudes toward health care in Britain. Many soldiers and civilians treated for bombing injuries received high-quality medical care for the first time in their lives, and they got it "free." The Beveridge Report of 1942, which advocated free and universal health services, was used in propaganda broadcasts during the war both to boost home morale and to persuade the enemy that the British system was superior. And the war was widely regarded as a triumph for state planning after two decades of economic stagnation—the specifically British depression of the 1920s and the worldwide depression of the 1930s. The success of the war effort made governmental provision of any service, even one as basic as health care, seem natural, proper, and efficient.[6] The nationalization of health care was just one part of a broad program of state ownership of basic industries promoted by the Labour government immediately after hostilities ended. But equally important, the NHS can be viewed as Britain's reward to itself after the sacrifices of war and before the privations of recovery.

Seven lean years followed the creation of the NHS, during which the proportion of gross national product devoted to health declined slowly. Privation was not confined to health care, however, for the British economy was recovering from wartime destruction and dislocations. Then ensued two robust, if not fat, decades lasting into the 1970s. NHS expenditures on health care rose steadily from 3.4 percent of gross national product in 1954 to 5.4 percent in 1978.[7] Health expenditures rose faster in other nations, but the increase in British outlays was enough to secure a steady improvement in quality.

But problems remained. Queues present at the start of the NHS did not disappear. British citizens, however, compared availability of care with what they had had before, not with the standards of other countries; and the continuing visits from wealthy foreigners to secure treatment showed that Britain provided some of the best health services in the world.

The typical British hospital remained Edwardian or older. The relative remuneration of physicians declined. But the number of admissions doubled, and the fruits of medical research transformed the character of medical care. In a class-ridden society, the NHS held out the promise of equal treatment before the class-blind threats of sickness and death. But this promise remained unfulfilled. Access was equalized, but use was not. According to some indicators, class differences in the use of health care and geographic variation in the availability of care remained almost as large in 1975 as they had been in 1948. But the NHS promised high-quality medical care to the acutely ill and increasingly delivered on that promise. It unquestionably spared patients the fear of financial ruin from medical bills. As a result, it became and remained one of the most popular institutions in Britain, second only to the Crown, and a close second at that.[8] The recent curtailment of the growth in health expenditures and the resulting stresses should be viewed against this background.

### How the National Health Service Works

Any health care system must solve two problems—how to ensure that patients are seen by the right health care providers, and how to pay for the services that providers render. The way the British system deals with these two issues differs sharply from the American approach.

## The Patient

Each British resident enrolls with one of approximately 27,000 general practitioners (GPs). Patients may choose any doctor who has an opening and may switch when they wish, but few exercise this option. A visit to a GP is normally the first point of contact with the health care system during any spell of illness. In the past, patients commonly stopped by to visit their GPs unannounced, but GPs are now trying to encourage their patients to make specific appointments. An office visit is likely to be brief, averaging six minutes. GPs carried an average of 2,200 patients in 1981.[9] If the patient is too ill to leave home, the GP will often make a house call. The GP may decide to prescribe medication or send specimens to hospital laboratories for analysis, but in most cases he cannot order complicated tests or admit patients to a hospital.

If the GP finds indications of an illness that requires more extensive testing or treatment than he can provide from his office, he will refer the patient to a consultant—a specialist, in American parlance. Nearly all specialists who see patients through the NHS are employed by regional health authorities on a salaried basis. The GP may write a letter to the consultant or telephone him. If the case is urgent, a call is likely to be made and the patient will be seen immediately. Otherwise, he may have to wait several weeks or even months for an appointment.

To avoid the usual waits, the patient may go directly to a hospital emergency room, a practice that is frequent enough to cause some concern about queue jumping. Or the GP may say that his patient is too ill to go to the consultant's office; in that event, the consultant will make a house call, generally after a much shorter delay. After examination, the consultant may prescribe further outpatient tests or treatment, schedule an admission to the hospital, or admit the patient immediately.

Patients on the waiting list are classified as urgent or nonurgent. Urgent cases are supposed to be admitted within one month and nonurgent cases within one year, but these standards are not met.[10] According to one correspondent, there are no objective definitions of which kinds of illness merit admission without delay; rather the distinction between such cases and others depends on the medical judgment of individual doctors and the availability of beds. The definitions of who should be on the waiting list vary from time to time and place to place.

For example, the criteria used for listing cases for immediate admission or for classifying them as urgent or nonurgent grew more exacting when a strike of hospital workers slowed admissions to a trickle and relaxed after the strike ended.

Waiting lists for admission to British hospitals are long. One-third of all admitted patients were on waiting lists for three months or more, 6 percent for one year or more. In March 1982 the waiting lists had 625,000 names. Nearly all the people on these lists were waiting for surgery, much of it elective in that delay does not threaten the patient's life.[11]

The size of these waiting lists clearly shows a demand for health care greater than supply. But the numbers are hard to interpret because the records on which they are based are poor. It is reported that patients may be listed for admission to several hospitals, that some deceased patients remain on lists, and that some are listed as waiting who really are not. For example, many patients whose names appear on waiting lists do not come in when they are called. Moreover, names of chronically ill patients appear on the lists even if they are merely awaiting further treatment at a fixed time. Similar problems hinder interpretation of data on waiting lists for treatment at outpatient clinics.[12] Despite these and other methodological problems, evidence is abundant that waiting times for specific treatments such as orthopedic surgery are very long, stretching into years in some regions.[13]

In sum, a British patient ordinarily has no direct access to a specialist through the NHS. Usually, he must first see a general practitioner. Only if his GP feels that the patient should see a consultant can he readily do so. Such sequential referral predated the NHS. British patients are reported to be using hospital emergency rooms increasingly to provide primary care. In emergency cases, waiting for hospital admission is rare.

By contrast, in the United States patients may see any doctor with whom they can get an appointment. Many physicians who provide primary care, such as routine checkups and examinations, also have specialist training. This difference between access to specialists in the United States and in Britain expresses national customs and attitudes about doctor-patient relations. British physicians, many of whom have studied or practiced in the United States, repeatedly told us that they think British patients are more likely than their American counterparts to accept a doctor's judgment as final. Part of the difference may come from a kind of New World prometheanism—American patients seem unwilling to acknowledge that there may be no effective therapy for certain illnesses.

Whatever the explanation, the British patient is clearly part of a structured social and medical care system, bound by custom and by a long-term dependency on his GP and conditioned to accept the authority of prestigious consultants. In contrast, the American patient is likely to see different doctors for different problems and more frequently to regard doctors as technicians who are periodically called on to repair his physical machinery, to be dropped if they are unable to solve the current problem or to be sued if they botched the last one.

### The System of Financial Support

The National Health Service is supported by government funds except for modest exceptions. Seventy-five percent of these funds come from general revenues. Another 20 percent come from earmarked involuntary contributions by each person covered under the NHS and from charges imposed for drugs, eyeglasses, and a few other items. And 5 percent come from other sources. About 60 percent of the British population is exempt from these charges for drugs and other items.[14]

Government provides health care through three channels that are administered by different government agencies. First, primary care is provided by general practitioners, who are employed by the NHS and who receive an income based on the number of patients they have and on whether they choose to practice in an area with a lower than specified physician-to-population ratio. The GP is also authorized to charge extra fees for special services. GPs may prescribe without budget limitations of any kind, except that prescription-happy doctors may come under review by other physicians and be warned. Both the salary of the GP and the cost of his prescriptions (excluding direct charges on the patient) are borne directly by the NHS. Legally, the GP can write a prescription for any drug, but in practice the power to prescribe has little financial reach because GPs provide patients no care more sophisticated (or costly) than that which can be dispensed from the office. Nevertheless, as the concern for limits on health budgets has continued and as the cost of drugs that can be prescribed by GPs has risen, the government has been forced to consider budget limits on the general practitioner service as well.[15]

Second, institutional care is provided through the system of hospitals and nursing homes of various kinds, organized in England in 192 districts and 14 regions. Such agencies allocate two-thirds of NHS expenditures. Scotland, Northern Ireland, and Wales each have separate health services and receive their budgets from the House of Commons.[16]

Third, nonhospital community care is provided by district nurses and health visitors, all under the administrative control of local authorities. The local authority is also responsible for social services, ambulance services, domestic help for the sick, and for the provision of some accommodation for the elderly who are not infirm enough to need a hospital bed. These services are financed by local authority budgets that are supported in part by local taxes and in part by payments from the central government.

Alongside government health services is a private health care system to be described below.

### Budget Setting

In the British system, with three exceptions, expenditures of all hospitals are limited by fixed budgets set by the national government.[17] Besides appropriated funds, British health institutions receive modest amounts of income from charity; from patients who use the small number of so-called pay beds in NHS facilities; and, in the case of some teaching hospitals, from endowments, mostly acquired before the creation of the NHS.

How do spending limits get set in Britain? Although the procedure is largely "top down," it is tightly constrained by spending levels in previous years. Each budget is formulated in the shadow of a published multiyear plan endorsed by the government. The British Treasury, which performs functions like those of the U.S. Office of Management and Budget, sets spending targets based on the previous year's outlays and anticipated inflation. It also determines whether the NHS will receive an increment for real growth in expenditures and, if so, how large it will be. The Treasury goes through similar exercises for other segments of public expenditure, and the full budget is ultimately modified and approved by the cabinet before being submitted to the House of Commons. In practice, party discipline assures that the House of Commons will not change the budget significantly.

The resulting health appropriation is a global projection for the

National Health Service. Thus the secretary of state for health and social services, the cabinet officer responsible for health and the NHS, retains some discretion in allocating expenditures among the fourteen health regions. The budget is divided into two parts, one part for new construction and capital equipment and the other for current operations; authority to move funds between these categories is strictly limited.[18]

Most funds are transferred successively from the Treasury to regions and districts. Decisions about equipment or services that will cover more than one district, such as blood banks, CT scanners, or coronary artery surgery, are determined nationally or regionally. Increases in the hospital medical staff require regional approval. Because the authorities believe that the best way to control the budget is to limit the number of hospital physicians, approval of new posts is hard to get.

Even the best-laid plans must sometimes be changed. When prices rise faster than anticipated, no adjustment is made in the current year and each jurisdiction must absorb the higher costs.[19] If any geographic entity overspends its budget, the excess is subtracted from its allocation for the next period. A second adjustment is made to account for movement of patients across jurisdictional boundaries. Each region is reimbursed an amount equal to its net "imports" multiplied by the average cost of patient care.[20] The arrangement compensates for patients who generate average costs but is inadequate for patients who leave their districts to get costly specialized care.

The effect of this system is roughly as follows. A hospital is likely to get a budget, adjusted for inflation, that is equal to that of the preceding year unless it can make a persuasive case for a specific additional outlay. If the cost of supplies or wages happens to rise more rapidly than the price index used by the health authorities for adjusting budgets, the hospital administrators and staff must find ways to cut back. Maintenance is an early casualty of restrictions on spending for current operations, with painting cycles, for example, sometimes stretching to decades. Long-term budget control depends on strictly enforced limits on the hiring of physicians, nurses, and other staff. Backlogs of requests for new equipment and replacement of old equipment grow—one piece of radiological equipment in a distinguished London hospital is approaching its golden anniversary.[21] The larger or more experimental the new expenditure, the more likely that the decision about it will be made at a higher jurisdiction, such as the region. A decision on whether to build a new hospital, for example, will fall in this category.

Because the total budget is fixed nationally, one locality can gain only at the expense of another. Only by stimulating charitable contributions can the creative local health official add to his own resources without reducing someone else's. Such gifts are small measured against total health expenditures, but have largely paid for some specialized new equipment.[22] Party discipline in Parliament helps the government enforce budget limits, and the inability of the regions and districts to obtain substantial funds from other sources assures that the limits will be binding.

The structure of governance within the hospital and the district also furthers the achievement of budget goals. The British hospital is a quasi-feudal enterprise, ruled largely by a peerage of senior physicians (consultants) who usually work only at one hospital and derive most or all of their income from salary. Each has junior physicians assigned to him, and each has a variable number of beds to which he can admit patients. British consultants are responsible, directly or indirectly, for the disposition of almost all the hospital's resources. The typical British hospital administrator, unlike his U.S. counterpart, has little power or authority within his institution. Thus consultants, whose personal salaries and positions are unaffected directly by budgetary vicissitudes, must parcel out the meager rations allotted through the health district. They have every incentive to do so amicably, for they are part of a select medical club whose members must work together, usually for the rest of their professional lives. That each has only a limited personal economic stake in the outcome of the allocations facilitates such cooperation.

Indeed, consultants who work part-time in the private sector may gain financially from tight NHS budgets. If patients move from the NHS, in which consultants work on fixed salary, to the private sector, the consultant who bills for his services is the gainer.

### Regional Inequalities

British health planners have tried to equalize expenditures among the regions. When the NHS began, parts of Britain had a number of new or endowed hospitals and an ample supply of physicians, but many other areas were much less fortunate. To improve the distribution of physicians, the NHS provided bonuses for general practitioners who set up practice in underserved areas. But until 1976 it made little progress in reducing the inequality of expenditure on hospital services across regions. In 1975 per capita spending in the highest-spending region was

39 percent higher than in the lowest-spending one, even after adjusting for the flow of patients across boundaries. Because pay scales in Britain are uniform (except for distinction awards), unlike those in the United States, they did not contribute to the disparities.[23] In any event, even in the mid-1970s this difference was nearly as great as when the NHS began.[24] Spending by the NHS may in fact understate variations in medical services, because regions with above-average spending also have most of the endowed voluntary hospitals that appear to have been disproportionate beneficiaries of charitable gifts.

In 1976 the Resource Allocation Working Party (RAWP) recommended the gradual elimination of regional differences in per capita expenditures, adjusted for medical need.[25] The lion's share of additional real resources was to go to the low-spending regions. Unfortunately, economic woes engendered by the recession of 1974 and 1975 forced a slowdown in the rate of growth of medical expenditures. From 1975 to 1982 growth of per capita medical expenditures (based on a general price deflator) was only 1.65 percent a year. Such growth was barely sufficient to cover the increased health requirements of an aging population. Thus achievement of the RAWP goals of boosting outlays in low-spending regions has been slowed by an aversion to cutting real outlays in high-spending regions.[26]

Some regional and subregional planners have tried to carry the policy of equalization from the fourteen regions to their districts. But a lack of information on movement of patients and other data makes it difficult to apply.[27] Furthermore, the goal of creating national or regional centers of excellence and the inappropriateness of offering complex care in sparsely populated places make equalization among the many, small districts undesirable. Critics of the RAWP plan claim that the same considerations make equalization undesirable at the regional level. The problem is how to balance conflicting goals: achieving equality of access against achieving efficiencies of scale and providing the high-technology, high-quality care and scientific advance that depend on concentration of resources.

### The Private Sector

Intertwined with the National Health Service is a private medical care system—vestigial or embryonic, depending on how one reads the future—that is not supported directly by the government. Aneurin Bevan, the Labour minister who fathered the initial legislation creating the NHS, overcame the opposition of the medical profession in part by promising that consultants employed by NHS hospitals could have a part-time private practice. Whether this arrangement was Bevan's Faustian pact with the devil or a farsighted compromise is still argued. Among the 455,000 acute care beds in NHS hospitals, there were about 2,800 "pay beds" in 1982 to which consultants might admit private patients.[28] Some pay beds are located in regular NHS wards; others are in separate wards or buildings. The hospitals charge private patients for the estimated cost of care, and the consultant bills the patient separately for his services, as is customary in the United States.

In 1981 private hospitals in England and Wales had 6,842 beds, making a total of nearly 10,000 beds for private care. Voluntary insurance covers roughly one-third of private hospital expenditures and one-quarter of the cost of private physicians' care.[29] British private hospitals have usually not had the range of services available in NHS hospitals—house staff or comprehensive laboratory services, for example. For this reason, private hospitals are not the preferred place of treatment for complex or risky surgery or serious illness.

Private outlays account for less than 5 percent of total expenditures on physicians and inpatient care and less than 12 percent of total medical expenditures.[30] But the private medical system plays a role far larger than the economic measures of its size. A person suffering from varicose veins, a hernia, or an arthritic hip, who finds intolerable the delay of a year or more before treatment through the NHS, can obtain care promptly in the private sector. Roughly half of all abortions are done privately.[31] Most private medicine is reported to occur around London and in other relatively well-to-do parts of Britain. Data on the proportion of NHS consultants in various regions who see patients privately support these reports.[32]

Patients may enter the private system at various points. A few choose to sign up with a private general practitioner.[33] More often patients elect to see a consultant privately either directly or after an initial referral by their NHS general practitioner. Thus a patient who is told that he must wait for treatment within the NHS may ask if he can obtain treatment more quickly from the consultant as a private patient. Or a patient facing a long wait for a bed in an aging NHS hospital may choose prompt treatment in a new private hospital or nursing home where he can have such amenities as a private room.

The smallness of the private sector more than three decades after the creation of the NHS testifies to the reservoir of popular satisfaction with the public system. But spectacular recent growth in the private sector shows the increasing dissatisfaction with some aspects of the NHS, caused largely by budget limits.

In 1980 private medical insurance covered 3.6 million people, only 6 percent of the population, but coverage rose nearly 60 percent between 1977 and 1980.[34] Insurance is an attractive fringe benefit that lets businesses assure key employees prompt service for elective care, allowing them to avoid the delays common to the NHS. Several unions also have sought health insurance coverage. The most celebrated is the Electrical and Plumbing Trades Union, whose members were first covered in 1979, but brewery workers in Birmingham and taxi drivers in London had negotiated coverage even earlier.[35]

Voluntary health insurance is inexpensive by U.S. standards for several reasons. First, almost all patients use their NHS general practitioner, even if they plan to see a consultant privately. Second, the NHS provides backup protection against serious complications: patients who require specialized care unavailable in private hospitals can be moved to an NHS facility. For example, if a major cardiac or pulmonary problem or a serious infection develops after hip surgery done in a private facility, the patient will be promptly transferred to a fully equipped NHS hospital. Third, the population covered by private insurance is usually employed and fairly young, and hence low risk. Fourth, British health care is less expensive than American care, in part because British doctors and other staff are paid less than their U.S. counterparts.[36]

Whether private medicine should be encouraged, shackled, or put out of existence is one of the most divisive issues facing British society and its policymakers. Is health care, like the obligation to vote or to bear arms during war, an attribute of citizenship to be regulated through political decisions? Is it a commodity like legal services or automobiles that should be allocated through the marketplace? Or is it a combination of the two? Michael Lee has characterized the difference between NHS medicine and private medicine in precisely these terms: "The private patient pays to avoid waiting; the NHS patient waits to avoid paying."[37]

There are two groups of issues involved in government policy toward private medicine. One concerns private medicine *within* the National Health Service, the question whether pay beds should be retained in NHS hospitals. After long controversy, the Labour government in 1976 began to eliminate them. But even in the decade before this decision, the number of pay beds in NHS hospitals had declined by about 22 percent, and occupancy rates were low.[38] In 1979 the Conservative government ended the policy of closing pay beds, arguing that the National Health Service gains if consultants do not have to leave NHS hospitals when they practice private medicine. But Labour has pledged to complete the elimination of private beds in NHS facilities when it returns to power.

As with most practical questions, the question of pay beds involves many principles—whether having pay beds helps NHS patients by siphoning off demand or hurts them by diverting resources such as trained nurses, whether consultants will provide care of the same quality to patients who pay them and to patients who do not, and whether the option of admitting patients to readily available pay beds causes consultants to delay admissions to NHS beds and thus to encourage patients to seek private care.

The second group of issues concerns private medicine *outside* the NHS. If the NHS continues to subsist within a budgetary straitjacket, private medicine is bound to continue growing, and controversy over the proper role for private medicine within a nationalized system will increase. Debates about whether the NHS subsidizes private medicine— by bearing the costs of training nurses or undercharging for pay beds— or whether private medicine subsidizes the NHS—by relieving the NHS of the cost of many patients—will intensify. The more NHS expenditures are curtailed, the more quickly government will be forced to develop a policy on how fast private health expenditures should be permitted to grow. It will have to decide not only whether to permit private hospitals to be built but whether to expand or shrink opportunities for NHS physicians to practice privately. For example, should government continue to allow NHS radiologists to use NHS facilities to perform CT scans for private patients? These and countless other issues will be the center of a battle between those who feel that health care is a right not to be sullied by markets and those who feel that markets should allocate some kinds of health care in some circumstances.

### Conclusions

At least seven features of the British health care system have facilitated the imposition of budget limits and made them stick. First, the

National Health Service is organized within a parliamentary democracy marked by party discipline; the House of Commons does not usually reverse policies set by the cabinet. Second, the principle of public ownership and management of important sectors of the British economy is widely accepted, particularly for health care services. Third, a reservoir of goodwill exists for the NHS because of its origins in wartime adversity and its assurance of care to even the poorest people. Fourth, sequential referral of patients—from general practitioner to consultant—creates a mechanism not present in the United States, which allows the trusted family doctor to screen out cases not deemed medically suitable for complex care. Fifth, the residue of class structure in Britain increases the ability of physicians to persuade patients that aggressive treatment is inappropriate and increases the willingness of patients to accept such bleak news. Sixth, the British are less driven than Americans by the "don't just stand there, do something" attitude toward disease. Finally, hospital governance by salaried consultants provides a notably effective instrument for encouraging the quiet enforcement of budget limits.

## part two

**Differences between U.S. and British Use of Technology**

*According to the ancient Greek philosopher Heraclitus, it is not possible to step into the same river twice. However brief the interval, the river will have changed. Much the same might be said of the modern hospital. The hospital patient of the 1980s may be diagnosed with the aid of equipment and treated with drugs and surgical procedures many of which did not exist as recently as a decade ago. He stays in the hospital for less time. He is served by many more staff—largely nurses and technicians—than he would have been ten years ago. And he will incur costs far more rapidly; the average cost per patient day in an American hospital was $288 in 1980, 3.7 times greater than in 1960 and 2.0 times greater than in 1970 after full account is taken of general inflation.*

*If one is looking for the effects of budget limits on health care, one should begin with their effects on the adoption of new technology. New diagnostic procedures and new methods of treatment must compete with established procedures for resources. In this part we describe how a contest has evolved with respect to several new methods of diagnosis and treatment. We also compare the provision of some traditional services that have undergone only modest change. Our description is intended to inform lay readers, not physicians or other experts who may find our presentation insufficiently detailed. The information we offer, though accurate, is intentionally presented in largely nontechnical terms. We observe that budget limits retarded the adoption of some, but not all, new procedures in Britain and in some instances led to levels of service far below those in the United States. Budget limits have also caused the British to provide less than the United States of some established procedures.*

*To provide the reader with an overview of what will follow in part 2, we can briefly summarize our findings as follows.*

*Three therapeutic procedures are provided at essentially the same level in Britain as in the United States.*

*1. All patients with hemophilia obtain high-quality treatment, including adequate supplies of the required clotting factors.*

*2. Megavoltage radiotherapy appears to be readily available in England to virtually all patients with cancer who can benefit from it.*

*3. Bone marrow transplantation is carried out with the same frequency per capita in Britain as in the United States.*

*Many other services are clearly rationed in Britain when compared with per capita levels of consumption in the United States.*

*1. The British carry out only half as many x-ray examinations per capita as Americans do, and they use only half as much film per examination.*

*2. The overall rate of treatment of chronic renal failure in Britain is less than half of that in the United States. Kidneys are transplanted at a comparable rate, but dialysis is carried out at a rate less than one-third of that in the United States.*

*3. Total parenteral nutrition is undertaken only about one-fourth as often in Britain as in the United States.*

*4. Great Britain has only one-sixth the CT scanning capability of the United States. Many major teaching hospitals lack a facility.*

*5. The British hospital system has only one-fifth to one-tenth as many intensive care beds, relative to population, as does the United States. Most hospitals have few intensive care beds or none at all.*

*6. The rate of coronary artery surgery in Britain is only 10 percent that of the United States. Even if the rate in the United States is excessive, the British could perform six or seven times more bypass procedures than at present, with probable benefit to patients.*

*7. Hip replacement is carried out three-quarters to four-fifths as often in Britain as in the United States.*

*Chemotherapy for cancer has, perhaps, an intermediate position between unrationed and rationed procedures. Chemotherapy for potentially curable tumors is administered at approximately the same rate as in the United States. On the other hand, tumors not highly responsive to chemotherapy are treated far less often.*

*The quality of British services in general is quite high, although shortages of personnel seem to have some deleterious effects on the quality of diagnostic x-ray and radiotherapy. Among the procedures that we studied, low investment appears to have substantial effect on the quality only of diagnostic radiology.*

*chapter three* **Matters of Life and Death**

Some of the most spectacular and costly advances in health care have yielded methods of keeping alive people who in the past would have died, often painfully. Chronic, severe kidney failure was fatal until machines were developed that substituted for many of the excretory functions of the kidney and techniques were developed for successfully transplanting kidneys. Hemophilia, the bleeding disease mentioned by history textbooks because it afflicted royal families, can now be treated so that patients, though never cured, can live almost normally. Cancer patients today are likely to be treated either by newly developed and costly drugs or hormones, some of which have proved effective against certain kinds of cancers and most of which were not available ten or fifteen years ago.

**Dialysis and Kidney Transplantation**

Kidney failure can occur either as the result of an injury from which the kidney can recover quickly or from damage that is progressive and irreversible. Severe kidney failure causes dangerous and potentially fatal accumulation of toxic wastes in the body fluids. By adjusting the diet, particularly the protein intake, the buildup of waste products can be slowed, but in chronic kidney failure the only definitive forms of treatment are dialysis and transplantation.

*Hemodialysis and Peritoneal Dialysis*

To carry out hemodialysis, blood is allowed to flow from the patient's artery through a machine where waste products diffuse through a thin membrane into a solution that is subsequently discarded. The cleansed blood is then returned to the patient's circulation through a vein. This process, which also removes any accumulated excess of fluid and salts, is usually carried out three times a week for four to five hours.

DIALYSIS IN CHRONIC IRREVERSIBLE KIDNEY FAILURE. Until the 1960s hemodialysis could be used only on a limited number of occasions because the repeated insertion of a tube progressively destroyed accessible blood vessels until no way of connecting the patient to the dialysis machine was available. Thus hemodialysis was not a practicable mode of treatment for patients with irreversible kidney failure. In the early 1960s a special shunt connecting artery and vein was developed that partially solved this problem.[1] Once inserted, this shunt can usually be left in place for six to nine months or more before such complications as clotting or infection force its removal. Later a technique was developed that permits an artery and a vein to be directly connected and the skin closed so that the body surface is left intact. Such a connection functions longer, is less unsightly than an external shunt, and has greatly facilitated the use of long-term hemodialysis.

The second method of removing waste products from the blood, peritoneal dialysis, requires placing a flexible plastic tube through the abdominal wall. A special dialysis solution is allowed to run into the abdominal cavity, and waste products plus excess water and salt move into the solution through the membrane that lines the abdominal cavity. At intervals, the fluid is drained from the abdomen and replaced with fresh solution.

The original technique for peritoneal dialysis proved useful primarily in acute, transient kidney failure. Its use in chronic kidney failure is limited because of the many hours that the patient must remain immobile each week and because of various complications, notably infections. A newer method, chronic ambulatory peritoneal dialysis (CAPD), permits the patient to be mobile and is also simple for the patient to use unaided. As a result CAPD is being applied to chronic renal failure more and more widely.

DIALYSIS IN ACUTE REVERSIBLE KIDNEY FAILURE. Acute reversible kidney failure is usually caused by shock or by medications that damage the kidney tubules. Urine flow falls to low levels or ceases for periods ranging from a few days to two or three weeks. In many such cases, dialysis is lifesaving, and its benefits are very large relative to the direct cost of several thousand dollars.

No statistics are available on the treatment of acute kidney failure in Britain, but according to experienced nephrologists, almost all patients have access to appropriate care. Peritoneal dialysis, which can be carried out in even the smallest hospital, is usually an effective form of therapy but, when hemodialysis is required, the patient can usually be transferred to a hospital that has the necessary facilities. The care of acute kidney failure in Britain, as with other acute illnesses, thus seems to approximate U.S. care. Furthermore, dialysis, once undertaken, is apparently carried out at a level of sophistication and staffing comparable to that in the United States.

DIALYSIS IN CHRONIC KIDNEY FAILURE. Although dialysis is literally the difference between life and death for patients with severe, irreversible kidney damage who cannot undergo successful transplantation, it is an imperfect substitute for normally functioning kidneys. The death rate of patients on dialysis under age fifty is 10 percent a year, and among older patients, 20 percent a year.[2] Moreover, a variety of problems impair the quality of life of the survivors. First, patients must spend many hours a week in treatment. Second, even with the best dialysis techniques patients continue to have metabolic problems and to be troubled by one or another symptom, such as itching of the skin, impotence, depression, insomnia, and easy fatigability.

### Transplantation

Transplantation has the great advantage that, if successful, it not only frees the patient from the travails of dialysis but also gives him a sense of complete good health. Transplantation is feasible, however, only if the patient is a suitable candidate for surgery and if a kidney can be found that his body can be induced not to reject. The kidney may be transplanted from a living donor (people normally have two kidneys but can usually manage with one) or from someone whose kidney was obtained promptly after death. Unless the patient has a blood relative (ideally a sibling) who is willing to donate a kidney, it is necessary to use a cadaver kidney. Only rarely does a nonrelated, living donor offer any immunologic advantage over a cadaver.

Patients over the age of about sixty are usually not considered suitable for transplantation because they have a high incidence of serious complications after surgery. Younger patients may also have medical problems, such as cancer, which make them unsuitable candidates. And some physicians are reluctant to let go a patient whose dialysis program they are supervising.

Except for identical twins, virtually all patients receiving a kidney must undergo therapy with drugs designed to prevent the body from rejecting the transplanted organ. Unfortunately, these drugs are not always effective in preventing rejection, with the result that nearly 40 percent of all kidneys transplanted from cadavers and almost 20 percent of kidneys transplanted from living related donors are rejected by the body and fail within one year.[3]

Both British and U.S. physicians remark on the failure to make use of potentially transplantable kidneys, largely because physicians to the terminally ill are loath to bring up the subject of donating organs and because it is difficult to arrange for kidneys to be transported from one area to another.

Finally, an important new development should be noted, the recent advent of cyclosporine. This powerful immunosuppressive agent dramatically reduces the incidence of serious infections and improves the results of organ transplantation.

### Cost of Treatment

Dialysis is not only trying but also expensive. In 1979 the annual charge for hemodialysis per patient in the United States was about $25,000 in hospitals and about $20,000 in dialysis centers (87 percent of all dialysis in the United States is done in hospitals or centers); the annual cost was about $15,000 if hemodialysis was done at home with the aid of friends or relatives.[4] The cost of hemodialysis in Britain in 1977 averaged $18,000 in hospitals and $11,500 at home.[5]* The cost of transplantation and follow-up treatment for one year is similar to the annual cost of home dialysis. In sharp contrast to the practice in the United States and almost all other countries, two-thirds of dialysis in Britain is done at home.[6] At recent exchange rates, dialysis is cheaper in Britain than in the United States, presumably because doctors, nurses, and technicians are paid less in Britain.

### Rates of Treatment

The most striking difference between British and U.S. treatment is that virtually every patient suffering from chronic kidney failure is

---

* Throughout the book we use exchange rates that correspond to the appropriate year.

treated in the United States, whereas most in Britain are not. The number of patients treated conveys the dimension of the difference. In the United Kingdom, 69 people per million were undergoing dialysis and 56 people per million had functioning transplants in 1980. By contrast, 230 people per million were undergoing dialysis in the United States in 1980 and about 57 per million are estimated to have had functioning transplants. In other words about one-fourth of American patients with total failure of their own kidneys had functioning transplants. Thus the proportion of the population undergoing dialysis in the United States is more than three times larger than that in the United Kingdom, and the proportion with functioning transplants is almost identical.[7]

### Financial Influences

The rate of dialysis in the United States is high because patients have been almost fully relieved of the cost of treatment, and physicians have been assured full reimbursement for all costs they incur. The federal government assumed this burden in 1972 through the end-stage renal disease program mandated under medicare. This program has encouraged center dialysis because it pays for out-of-pocket costs up to a set maximum fee that covers all costs at centers, including a payment to the physician for each visit. By contrast, no reimbursement is provided for the time and inconvenience of friends or relatives who help a patient on home dialysis. Thus there has been no financial reason for nephrologists to encourage the patient to seek a transplant or home dialysis, and patients have had no financial incentive to seek home care.

In sharp contrast, dialysis in Britain must compete with other health services for financing, and hospital dialysis must compete for limited hospital space. The consultant nephrologist, to whom general practitioners and other hospital-based physicians refer cases of kidney failure, must secure hospital space, obtain dialysis machines, and get permission to hire and train nurses and technicians to run them. Machines themselves have not been a bottleneck.

Implementing a home dialysis program is easier than starting or enlarging a center, because it requires neither scarce hospital space nor day-to-day supervision by skilled nursing personnel. Nurses are necessary only to train the patient and family. The friends or relatives who help patients with dialysis at home are not paid by the National Health Service, and the bedroom or other space where dialysis is performed does not crowd out other NHS activities. Once a patient has been trained in home dialysis, the principal direct cost is dialysis fluids and other sterile supplies. Because of the system's commitment to clinical freedom, each doctor can draw on such supplies without explicit budget limitation. One energetic nephrologist was able to increase the resources effectively at his disposal by pushing home dialysis. He thus acquired roughly $200,000 a year in sterile supplies, partly circumventing the limit on personnel, equipment, and hospital space. As one consultant nephrologist put it, "I must create propaganda in my unit which puts pressure on patients not to get stuck on the limited hospital dialysis facilities but to submit themselves and their families to the incessant demands of home dialysis or to submit themselves and their families for transplantation."[8]

### Limiting Treatment in Britain

If so many fewer cases of kidney failure are being treated in Britain than in the United States and other countries, who is not being treated and how are decisions on treatment made? Age is clearly a factor. Up through age forty-four the rate at which new patients are accepted for treatment is the same in Britain as in France, West Germany, and Italy. Among patients forty-five through fifty-four the rate of treatment in Britain is about two-thirds of the rate in those three countries; among patients fifty-five through sixty-four, about one-third; and among patients sixty-five or older, less than one-tenth.* There are, however, many reasons, other than age, that may cause a patient to be rejected. Patients with vascular complications of diabetes figure prominently among those considered unsuitable for treatment in Britain. Other medical diseases, physical handicaps, and mental illness also seem to be common reasons for rejection. People who carry hepatitis are also viewed unfavorably, because they must be treated in segregated areas at great additional expense. The lack of adequate facilities for home dialysis is also a common reason for not accepting a patient. By contrast, in the United States and in Western Europe most patients with such impediments to treatment are accepted for dialysis or transplantation. Indeed, even in

---

* Other developed industrial countries have rates of dialysis that range between the U.S. and British rates. In Britain 111 cases of renal failure per million population were being treated in 1979; the corresponding numbers for selected other countries were France, 188; Federal Republic of Germany, 161; Netherlands, 149; Sweden, 150; and Switzerland, 221. *Combined Report on Regular Dialysis and Transplantation in Europe, X, 1979* (Basel; Hospal, Ltd., 1979), p. 4.

Britain, it appears that no patient with any one of the criteria of unsuitability just listed would be rejected by all dialysis units. In other words, the criteria for rejection varied widely from center to center.[9]

CRITERIA FOR REJECTION. Resource constraints, rather than medical criteria, are largely responsible for the lower rate of dialysis in Britain, though some British physicians still dispute this conclusion. The *Lancet*, one of the two leading British medical journals, stated in an editorial column in 1981 that "chronic dialysis is a resource which is necessarily limited. Lines, therefore, have to be drawn and they are seen to be drawn. The chosen have their life-saving treatment: the rest do not and they and their relatives probably know it."[10] The view that resource constraints are the key to decisions about whom to dialyze gains further support from the finding that criteria for acceptance differ from region to region. Rates of acceptance clearly correlate with the variable resources allocated to renal failure. To some extent these regional differences are traceable to the origins of the dialysis program in Britain. The capital costs of the first dialysis units came directly from the Department of Health and Social Security, though operating expenses had to be met by the regions. Most units were placed in academic centers, a pattern that has persisted. As a result, Greater London has ten or eleven centers, while the West Midlands, with 40 percent of London's population, has only two.[11]

It is easy, moreover, to imagine that conscientious doctors, confronted with the continual frustration of having to turn patients away, might fashion criteria that justified a refusal to treat. Sometimes, however, such rationalizations fail, and the doctor faces a real dilemma. What about the sixty-year-old patient without any evidence of cancer, or of vascular or other systemic disease, who now develops chronic renal failure? If he is in full possession of his faculties and productive at his work, what reason can be found to refuse him treatment? Many such patients are under treatment in the United States, but few in Britain. An English consultant in a large community hospital had a ready answer. Everyone over fifty-five, he said, is "a bit crumbly" and therefore not really a suitable candidate for therapy.

THE PHYSICIANS' ROLE. Some responsible physicians still refuse to acknowledge resource constraints as an element of decisionmaking. The Medical Services Study Group of the Royal College of Physicians, from an extensive audit of records of patients under fifty, reported in the *British Medical Journal* in 1981 that the reasons given for nonacceptance were sound and that no patient was denied dialysis because of inadequate facilities. This conclusion drew heavy fire. An accompanying editorial noted the strong correlation between availability of facilities and numbers of patients treated, suggesting that the distribution of facilities does not match the distribution of renal failure. The editorialist also pointed out the flaw in considering only patients under fifty, because only this cohort receives treatment in near adequate numbers. Others, in letters to the editor, put forth various weak excuses—for example, "the patient spoke no English"—as the reason for rejection.[12]

There remains, however, one oddity that, on the surface, would suggest that no shortage of facilities exists. When queried in 1980, most dialysis unit directors reported that they were "coping with demand."[13] In fact they were treating almost all referred patients judged suitable for dialysis by the directors' own medical criteria. How can dialysis centers avoid congestion when the number of candidates for dialysis vastly exceeds capacity? Only one director indicated that he was rejecting good, rather than borderline, cases.

The answer seems to lie with the expectations and the resulting referral patterns of general practitioners and physicians in the internal medicine departments of the local hospitals. From discussions with such doctors, we found that they quickly become attuned to the criteria that lead to a patient's acceptance by the center. No advantage accrues to anyone if the local physician flouts these norms and refers "unsuitable" patients. The nephrologist must then tell the patient and family that treatment is not available, or he must contradict the referring internist and say the patient is not an appropriate candidate. The referring physician must admit to error in the referral or acknowledge that resource constraints preclude treatment. The family and patient, in turn, will be far more upset than if they were told initially that dialysis and transplantation were not appropriate because of the overall medical picture. Little wonder that the local internist learns to strike a balance between medical indications and resource realities. Little wonder, too, that as more resources become available, a new balance is struck between demand and supply.

British physicians are candid about the way they discourage patients from insisting on dialysis. Asked how he would explain to her family the prospects of a sixty-five-year-old woman with kidney failure, one general practitioner first told us that he did not think it was up to him to decide whether she should be dialyzed, that he would leave the decision to the consultant. But then he added, "Obviously the patient is sixty-five and therefore does not come within the regional dialysis program." When pressed on whether he might save everyone time and anguish by discouraging referral, he described how he would talk to the family. "I would say that mother's or aunt's kidneys have failed or are failing and there is very little that anybody can do about it because of her age and general physical state, and that it would be my suggestion or my advice that we spare her any further investigation, any further painful procedure and we would just make her as comfortable as we can for what remains of her life." Remarkably, few of the criteria for rejection are explicitly stated. Age, for example, is not officially identified as an obstacle to treatment.

To summarize, the process by which British patients are denied treatment is rooted in resource limits. But clearly many British physicians feel that even with unlimited resources they would not treat some kidney patients who would be treated in the United States, such as those with long-standing diabetes with its devastating effects. As one consultant stated, "I think that you should prolong life, but you should not prolong dying."

Because of the respect that most patients have for physicians, the recommendation of the doctor is usually followed with little complaint, particularly when the disease does not manifest itself in a way that is recognizable to the patient or when it is only one manifestation of a multifaceted disorder like diabetes.

### Hemophilia

In contrast to patients with severe kidney problems, almost all hemophiliacs diagnosed in Britain are treated. Unlike kidney failure, which largely strikes older adults, hemophilia usually becomes apparent in childhood. (Mild hemophiliacs may not be diagnosed until later in life, when an event, such as surgery, uncovers the disease.) If patients are not treated by modern methods, most will die young after increasingly painful and immobilizing episodes of internal bleeding.

#### Nature of the Disease

Hemophilia is an uncommon disease, usually genetic in origin. The defect is carried without symptoms by the mother and transmitted, on the average, to half her sons. Hemophilia is a single name for two

diseases characterized by the partial or complete absence of either of
two components of normal blood—factor VIII and factor IX, both of
which promote clotting. Insufficiency of factor VIII is called hemophilia
A; that of factor IX is called hemophilia B, or Christmas disease, so
named after the first diagnosed patient. Apparently no one suffers from
both variants of the disease. Contrary to popular myth, the scourge of
the hemophiliac is not the cut or bruise from which he bleeds to death.
Rather, the hemophiliac suffers periodic internal hemorrhages that may
follow a bruise or happen spontaneously. Bleeding usually occurs in
joints, but it may occur in muscles, the kidneys, and, in rare but dangerous
cases, the head. Bleeding damages, and repeated bleeding may destroy,
the joint in which it occurs.

The onset of an episode is usually marked by tingling or warmth and
may be accompanied by restlessness or anxiety. Within a few hours mild
discomfort and restriction of motion may follow. Next come pain,
swelling, skin warmth, and severe limits on motion. After a period
ranging from days to weeks, the blood that caused the symptoms is
resorbed.

In all cases early treatment is likely to be most effective in reducing
short-term discomfort and long-term damage. The untreated hemophiliac
can look forward to increasingly frequent and painful attacks, progressive restriction of movement, and to a life that, to paraphrase Hobbes,
is nasty, brutish, and short.

Hemophilia may be classified as severe, moderate, or mild, according
to the proportion of the normal endowment of factor VIII or factor IX
that is missing. Of greater importance is the frequency of hemorrhage,
which largely depends on the age, activities, and previous treatment of
the patient rather than on the precise deficiency of one of the factors.
Severe hemophiliacs average about one bleeding episode a week; somewhat over half of all patients suffer from severe hemophilia, and more
than four-fifths of these have hemophilia A.[14]

### Treatment

Until the late 1960s hemophilia A could be treated imperfectly and
only by the cumbersome method of transfusing with plasma. Because a
unit of normal plasma contains only a small amount of factor VIII or
factor IX, and because patients can tolerate only a limited volume of
fluids by transfusion, it was not possible to add enough of the missing
blood factor to achieve good results. Consequently, hemophiliacs re-

quired frequent hospitalization and suffered from progressive deterioration of their joints.

During the second half of the 1960s, new techniques were developed to reduce the volume of each transfusion by using only the precipitate from frozen plasma. The availability of cryoprecipitate made it practical to administer large quantities of factor VIII in a small volume. Initially only a small quantity of this new blood product could be produced, and only the large medical centers had it. But concentrates of factor VIII became available in both the United States and Britain in the early 1970s. By the mid-1970s nearly all patients were entered into treatment programs. That the new concentrates did not have to be kept frozen also facilitated home therapy. At about the same time, concentrated factor IX became commercially available, and it became possible to treat hemophilia B effectively and easily.

### Dosage and Cost

When a patient suffers a bleeding episode, administration of factor VIII or factor IX will probably end the bleeding and associated discomfort. But the degree of success with the first dose and the speed with which the dose is effective are uncertain. Results depend on the size of the dose, the severity of the underlying disease, the age and previous treatment of the patient, and the speed with which medication is administered after the onset of an episode. To complicate matters still further, large doses are thought to increase somewhat the risk of abnormal liver function resulting from impurities in the blood samples from which the factors are obtained. Furthermore, both concentrates and cryoprecipitate are expensive. The cost of therapy depends sensitively on the price per unit of factor VIII or factor IX. The typical patient requires 20,000 to 40,000 units a year of the missing factor. Some patients, however, are far more costly to treat because they have developed antibodies that destroy the clotting factors and that must be neutralized before therapy is effective. Despite the fact that treatment in Britain is somewhat less intensive, the cost is higher than in the United States because the price of blood factors used in therapy is higher. The average cost of treating hemophiliacs at home was reported to be $5,600 in the United States in 1982 and $6,000 within the NHS in 1980.[15] Because optimal treatment is costly and remains subjective, the best method of treatment remains controversial.

On two questions of care, British and American physicians essentially agree. One is whether to treat patients episodically (that is, when a hemorrhage occurs) or prophylactically (that is, to reduce the frequency of bleeding by administering low doses of factor VIII and IX, typically every other day). Prophylactic treatment is much more expensive because it requires far more concentrate. It is used in only about 4 percent of all cases in both countries, but the fraction is reported to be increasing.[16] The other question is whether to treat episodes in specialized centers or to train people to administer the deficient factor to themselves at home. Physicians in both countries use the second method whenever possible because treatment can begin as soon as a patient senses the onset of a hemorrhage.

On how much factor VIII or cryoprecipitate people require, some difference remains between standard practices in Britain and the United States. The average U.S. patient receives about 50 percent more factor VIII concentrate or cryoprecipitate than do patients in Britain. But the difference lies within the range of clinical uncertainty, because the consequences of lower dosages have been the subject of few studies. Early work seemed to indicate that doses even lower than those now used in Britain would produce satisfactory results; a 1980 study by a British team indicated, however, that doses approximating those common in the United States are often more effective than smaller doses, though lower doses sometimes suffice. Practices vary among other countries as well. Doses in the United States, for example, are perhaps half as large as those in West Germany, but there is no evidence that the higher German dosages produce better results.[17]

Although views on optimal dosages vary, two facts are clear: first, all diagnosed patients in both Britain and the United States are treated to levels that their physicians think optimal; and second, most British physicians favor a less-intensive, lower-cost program of therapy than do American physicians. These differences are reported to be narrowing and may vanish soon. Doctors in Britain claim that medical considerations, rather than resource limits, dictate how they practice, and the medical evidence cannot refute this position.

### The Treatment of Cancer by Radiotherapy

Cancer is the second most frequent cause of death in both the United States and Britain. In 1979 an estimated 765,000 patients were diagnosed in the United States as having cancers other than skin cancer, and more than 403,000 died of the disease. In Britain the corresponding figures were 235,000 and 136,000.[18] Cancer is treated by three means: surgery, radiotherapy, and chemotherapy. The five-year survival rate for patients undergoing therapy is nearly 50 percent.[19]

Radiation therapy has as its goal the destruction of malignant cells, but it also damages normal tissues. The limit on treatment is set by the damage to normal tissues that patients can tolerate.

Machines used in radiation therapy vary in power. For potentially curable malignancies, other than skin cancer, ideal therapy requires expensive machines with an energy level greater than a million electron volts (MeV). The machines most widely used are either cobalt 60 units or linear accelerators in the 4 to 6 million volt range. Some linear accelerators and betatrons produce radiation ranging from 15 to 45 MeV. For palliation, rather than cure, smaller machines, usually of 300 kilovolt capacity, produce good results, but treatment with such low-voltage machines is far from ideal because they frequently cause serious skin damage.

### Quantity of Equipment

There is no shortage of megavoltage radiation equipment in the United States. Indeed, there may be too much. In 1977 the average annual case load per high-energy unit was about 235, whereas each machine could readily handle 500 patients. Thirty percent of units operated below the guideline for minimal use—300 patients, or about 5,000 treatments a year—defined by the Health Resources Administration.[20] Part of the explanation for this "surplus" lies in the low population density of many parts of the United States; as a result, some machines are used below capacity to avoid patients' spending excessive time traveling to and from treatment.

Britain has only 44 percent as many megavolt machines available per capita.[21] Nevertheless Britain has enough megavoltage equipment to treat all patients with potentially curable cancer and those who require palliation. This conclusion derives from the following analysis: 117,000 patients were treated with radiotherapy in Britain in 1977. Of these, we estimate that 19 percent were treated for skin cancer, leaving a total of about 95,000 systemic cancers, or about 1,700 cases per million population, slightly more than in the United States. Assuming an average number of sixteen treatments per patient, as in the United States, these patients would require an aggregate of 1.5 million treatments. Because the British have 162 megavoltage machines, each capable of providing 10,000 treatments a year, there is a capacity of 1.6 million treatments. Indeed, with some effort, 12,000 treatments a year could be achieved on each machine, which would provide a substantial excess of supply over demand.[22]

Even this analysis may depict a less favorable picture than actually exists in Britain. Information from a leading British radiotherapist indicates that the U.S. figure of sixteen treatments per case is considerably higher than is thought appropriate and than is used in Britain.[23] Regional variations in the availability of equipment may result in some local shortages in Britain, but this problem is unlikely to be serious or widespread.

### Quality of Equipment

The United States has slightly better equipment and many more radiotherapists and physicists, but far fewer radiotherapy technicians (called radiographers in Britain) than does Britain.[24] The age and other characteristics of U.S. and British megavoltage equipment are similar, except that the United States has proportionately more machines that deliver over 10 MeV. Even so, the United States has relatively few high-energy machines because they are costly and there is considerable dispute about the additional benefits they confer. High-energy accelerators in the 10 to 20 MeV range cost about twice as much as units in the 4 to 6 MeV range.[25]

All experts agree that, other things equal, very high energy machines deliver a given dose of radiation to tumors with less damage to normal tissues than smaller machines do. But the practical importance of the difference is in dispute. Some therapists argue that perhaps 30 to 50 percent of patients can benefit from the use of the big machines, not because the cure rate with them is higher, but rather because complications are fewer and morbidity is reduced.[26] Other equally reputable therapists hold that the theoretical advantages of large machines do not show up in practice and that doctors can accomplish virtually the same results with 4 to 6 MeV units if they plan treatment with particular care. Indeed, no study convincingly demonstrates that higher morbidity and more complications result from the use of the low-energy machines. For this reason, some experts deny that the big, costly accelerators are worth what they cost.

Given this dispute, the British decision to buy few high-energy, high-cost machines is easy to understand, and we have no reason to believe that it has appreciably degraded the quality of care.[27]

### Staff

Effective therapy requires sufficient staff—radiotherapists, radiotherapy technicians, and physicists—to plan and execute therapy. A shortage of radiotherapists or physicists means either that patients can spend little time with their doctors or that therapy must be hastily or imprecisely planned. A shortage of technicians imposes excessive burdens on those charged with actually providing care.

A report to the National Cancer Institute recommends that there be at least one radiotherapist for each 200 to 250 new patients seen a year. The United Kingdom, with one radiotherapist for every 288 patients, does not meet this standard, but the United States has a fully acceptable staffing level, with one radiotherapist for 177 patients.[28] There should also be two to three technologists for each megavoltage machine and one for each heavily used kilovoltage machine.[29] Britain easily meets these standards, but the United States does not.[30] American experts acknowledge a shortage of radiotherapy technologists. This shortage means that American radiotherapists and physicists carry out more actual treatment than their counterparts do in Britain.

In the aggregate, the British cancer treatment centers have about 40 percent fewer physicists than would be optimal, whereas the United States is apparently adequately staffed. The shortage of physicists is not apparent at large British cancer centers, but in 1981 the chairman of the physicists' association reported gross understaffing in some units.[31]

### Conclusions

The per capita quantity of radiotherapy in Britain is almost identical with that in the United States. Demand for care in both countries is being fully met. This conclusion is consistent with the expressed views of British radiotherapists, who told us that all patients can be promptly accommodated in one or another treatment center.

But the quality of care may be marginally lower in Britain. The modest difference in quality derives not from the type or age of available machines but from differences in staffing. The number of radiotherapists in Britain is below the minimal recommended value. And the availability in Britain of only half as many physicists per new patient as in the United States has, in the opinion of experts, some appreciable effect on quality. Shortages of professional staff also curtail the time spent on research, teaching, and continued education.

On the other hand, Britain has far more radiotherapy technicians per patient than the United States does, more even than the U.S. target. From this fact we conclude, and experts confirm, that radiotherapy technicians in Britain carry out some of the tasks done by radiotherapists and physicists in the United States. Such an arrangement is not optimal, but we have no data on how large the loss may be. This staffing pattern is not surprising given the resource constraints of the British health care system. Substituting technicians for more expensive personnel, providing there is only a slight loss of quality, makes sense when other sectors of the system are starving for funds.

The situation is very different in the United States. Because technicians are in short supply, they are often rushed and work under excessive stress. Low salaries caused by wage rigidity, rather than resource constraints, are at the heart of the U.S. problem.

The fairly complete treatment of cancer in both countries is remarkable given the age of patients. Most patients over fifty-five are denied chronic dialysis in Britain, but they are not denied radiotherapy.

It should be emphasized, of course, that radiotherapy costs only $500 million a year in the United States and probably much less than $125 million in Britain. The British population is about one-fourth of the U.S. population, but, as noted, the British medical salary structure is lower and British centers on average use their radiotherapy equipment nearer to capacity than do American centers. Thus the British could not save much by reducing the quality and quantity of radiotherapy treatment.

### Cancer Chemotherapy

The treatment of cancer with chemotherapeutic agents is growing rapidly. Agents developed during the last ten to fifteen years have made possible the cure of some patients with metastatic tumors that previously were almost always fatal. The dozen or so disorders in which the outlook has changed dramatically include advanced Hodgkin's disease, testicular carcinoma, acute lymphatic leukemia in childhood, and certain other childhood tumors. In the United States one-third to two-thirds of patients with these diseases and 90 percent of those with testicular cancer now enjoy long-term complete remissions. In the aggregate, however, such tumors comprise only a small percent of the total number of otherwise fatal cancers. Drug therapy can prolong useful life in approximately 92,000 of the 200,000 patients with metastatic disease. Of the 92,000, only 32,000 have cancers that are now potentially curable with drugs.[32]

Roughly thirty cytotoxic drugs are commercially available. They act by inhibiting DNA or RNA synthesis within cells and thus reduce the capacity of the cells to proliferate. These agents act in different ways. Some closely resemble substances normally metabolized by cells but differ enough to disrupt normal cell growth. Others inhibit the division of cells and thus limit multiplication. The ideal chemotherapeutic drug would attack only the tumor. But no drug is ideal. All the commercially available drugs harm normal cells to some degree and therefore cause toxic side effects. Side effects are of two kinds, acute and long term. About half of all patients, for example, suffer nausea and vomiting, which is sometimes very severe during the few days of treatment each month. Long-term effects are quite different. The most frequent are loss of hair, diminished appetite, weight loss, diarrhea, and fatigue that is sometimes nearly disabling. As a result, most agents markedly impair the quality of life of many patients.

Life-threatening complications are uncommon. The most frequent is suppression of bone marrow function, with a resulting drop in the number of white blood cells or platelets. The patient with too few white blood cells is susceptible to infection, sometimes of overwhelming severity. If the number of platelets is sharply reduced, bleeding into the skin, gastrointestinal tract, or other organs may occur, a potentially fatal but treatable complication. Fortunately, the physician can usually detect changes in blood counts before they become severe and can deal with them by adjusting doses or changing drugs. Other serious conditions, such as damage to the liver, heart, kidneys, and lungs also occur, but only infrequently.

Some metastatic tumors can be treated by endocrine therapy—either by removing an organ that produces a tumor-stimulating hormone or by administering large doses of hormone that inhibit tumor growth. This form of treatment, used most often in carcinoma of the breast and of the prostate, commonly produces a remission of the disease or a palliation of symptoms but rarely effects a cure.

Various forms of treatment designed to influence the body's immune mechanisms have also been used, but success has been limited. Recently, however, antibodies have been produced that seek out specific tumor cells and destroy them. Such experimental work may bring about notable changes in the treatment of some cancers.

### Treatment in the United States

Approximately four-fifths of cancer treatments occur either in physicians' offices or in hospital outpatient clinics. The patient will usually see the physician as often as twenty to thirty times a year at a cost of perhaps $50 a visit and will undergo x-ray examinations costing $500 to $1,000 a year. The total cost per ambulatory patient ranges from $2,000 to $2,500 annually. On the basis of expert estimates that 200,000 to 300,000 patients a year receive chemotherapy, the total cost of ambulatory care, excluding chemotherapeutic agents, would be $250 million to $500 million annually.[33] If an estimated 50,000 patients require six days of hospitalization at $500 a day, this portion of care costs $150 million a year.

The drug bill for chemotherapeutic agents in the United States in 1981 was $250 million: $200 million was spent on hospital and ambulatory patients and $50 million was spent by the National Cancer Institute on clinical trials.[34] The total cost of chemotherapy is therefore roughly $650 million to $900 million a year ($250 million for drugs, $250 to $500 million for outpatient care, and $150 million for hospital care).

Optimum chemotherapy requires an adequate number of trained oncologists and supporting staff and access to laboratory and x-ray services. The United States is well endowed with medical and pediatric oncologists; there were more than 3,000 in 1980.[35] It also has an adequate supply of oncology nurses and sufficient facilities to provide routine laboratory and x-ray services.

Oncologists deal with four groups of patients. The first comprises those who have a good chance of being cured. They make up about 5 percent of the total cancer population. Essentially, all such patients receive treatment.

For a second group of patients with metastatic disease, treatment alleviates symptoms. In breast cancer and in prostatic cancer, hormonal therapy with estrogen (or certain estrogen analogues) produces striking relief of symptoms, most notably bone pain. In patients with breast cancer, hormonal therapy may also extend life briefly. Therapy for both diseases is inexpensive and produces few side effects. For these reasons, active intervention is undertaken almost routinely. In patients with certain solid tumors, such as those of the lung, pancreas, colon, and stomach, chemotherapy often relieves symptoms.

The third group of patients with metastatic disease consists of patients who are not candidates for palliative therapy because they have few symptoms. In some such cases, chemotherapy may reduce tumor size and increase life expectancy, but it rarely effects a cure. Ovarian and small-cell lung carcinoma are examples of diseases in which life is often extended for as much as several years. Benefits in these cases clearly outweigh the side effects that commonly occur. The response to treatment in most other solid tumors is less clear. In a small number of patients life may be extended for a few months, but only at the cost of many side effects and complications in the group as a whole. The tumor often shrinks, but this response does not necessarily mean that life will be appreciably prolonged.

A final group of patients, free of apparent metastases after surgical removal of the tumor, receives so-called adjuvant chemotherapy to destroy remaining small, undetectable groups of tumor cells. Adjuvant chemotherapy cures some childhood cancers and extends the lives of some patients with breast cancer. But in most patients with breast cancer, as well as in those with other malignant diseases, the value of adjuvant therapy remains unproved and controversial.

### Treatment in Britain

Britain spent approximately $18 million on chemotherapeutic agents in 1981,[36] about 70 percent less than the United States on a population-corrected basis. Statements from British and U.S. physicians who have practiced in both countries confirm the implication of these statistics: chemotherapy is used much less frequently in Britain than in the United States. The British deal promptly with treatable metastatic tumors and apply the same procedures as here.[37] Palliation of prostatic and breast carcinoma is also carried out routinely. In these cases, practices in the United States and Britain appear similar.

In several respects British treatment of patients with metastatic disease differs markedly from U.S. treatment. Some British experts report that adjuvant chemotherapy is used only in pediatric cases and in breast cancer, and not all experts believe that the evidence supports the use of adjuvant therapy even in those cases. Oncologists with experience in both countries estimate that, in general, the rate of treatment of solid tumors in Britain is only one-fifth or one-sixth as high as in the United States. Data on the volume and types of drugs used in Britain support this conclusion. By linking information on drug regimens used for different types of cancer in Britain with statistics on the amount of each cancer chemotherapeutic agent sold in that country in 1981, we found that tumors such as those of the colon, pancreas, and stomach are not often treated.[38]

The lower rate of drug use in Britain implies far smaller expenditure on chemotherapeutic management. Using the estimate we made for the cost of physician services, x-rays, and laboratory costs in the United States, we calculate that the British provide chemotherapy that would cost $50 to $75 million in the United States. Because the cost of producing services is lower in Britain, actual expenditure is $30 to $45 million, against the $650 to $900 million spent in the United States. Thus, on a per capita basis, the British spend only about one-fifth as much as do Americans.

### Reasons for the Differences in Treatment

Why is treatment of incurable metastatic cancer so much more widespread in the United States than in Britain? Neither the method of financing treatment nor the cost of drugs can explain the difference. In both countries patients bear few direct monetary costs at the time of treatment. The National Health Service in Britain and private insurance and other third-party payment in the United States insulate patients from the cost of treatment. Moreover, under the rubric of "clinical freedom" the British physician can order whatever pharmaceuticals seem to him appropriate. Cost thus limits the number of patients treated only under the unusual circumstance in which the drug budget of a hospital gets so out of hand that it threatens the funding of other services. Under such circumstances, as at one of Britain's leading oncology centers, peer pressure is used to control the problem.

If costs are not the key factor in limiting treatment, what is responsible? For one thing, many British and some American oncologists doubt that the treatment of most metastatic solid tumors is medically justified. According to one British oncologist, "Apart from certain rare tumors—for instance leukemias, lymphomas, and choriocarcinoma—there is little hard evidence to show that the duration of life of a good quality is usefully extended. . . . The skeptically noncommited oncologist instinctively feels that the problems associated with chemotherapeutic combinations far outweigh the dubious benefits."[39] Other British oncologists expressed similar opinions to us. One stated, "Many of us would contend that the quality of life of many patients with metastatic cancer is improved by not having to suffer treatment which brings them nothing but unpleasant side effects and is of no benefit to them. . . . The main difference between American and British practice is that Americans tend to assume that treatment will do people good and we tend to assume that for many solid tumors it will not do so and that, furthermore, the handful of patients who will benefit will only do so marginally." Another said, "It is generally not considered worthwhile treating all patients with potentially toxic therapy for the sake of a temporary tumor regression in 20 percent of patients with doubtful survival improvement." Still another British oncologist told us that the "United States is squandering large sums of money on ineffective treatment."

Although many American oncologists argue that everything possible should be done, even if only a tiny chance exists to improve or extend life, some agree with the views just cited. For example, a leading American authority tersely asserted, "For many of the more common solid tumors there is no evidence that chemotherapy does any tangible good, regardless of the stage of the disease."[40] One British oncologist told us that U.S. physicians "confuse activity with progress" and wryly noted that for U.S. patients "it is becoming increasingly hard to escape chemotherapy."

Treatment is also more frequent in the United States because magazines, newspapers, and television trumpet each new advance in chemotherapy. Desperate patients, knowing that some drug is available, press hard for active intervention. Patients go directly to any of an ample supply of oncologists. The fee-for-service system in the United States provides still another incentive. Oncologists make their living by treating cancer; they naturally view chemotherapy in a rosier light than would people not dependent for their incomes on an activist approach.

The situation in Britain is quite different. Patients there are reported to be less knowledgeable than U.S. patients and to press less hard for intervention if their hospital consultant does not recommend it. Further-more, there are only forty to fifty consultants in oncology and hematology in all England and Wales, less than one-tenth as many as in the United States per capita.[41] Moreover, we were told, officials are reluctant to create new posts because of the increased expenditures on care that would inevitably result.

One British expert also suggested that, though no one with a potentially curable cancer is now denied treatment, the situation could change if an expensive, highly effective therapy suddenly became available for the treatment of one of the common forms of cancer. If such a treatment for cancer of the colon or cancer of the stomach were discovered, it would impose a considerable new financial burden on the health care system. One prominent oncologist said that he "wakes up screaming at such a prospect" and expressed the opinion that not everyone would be treated. Age, he indicated, might be used to determine who receives therapy, because curing a young person would secure more good years of life than would a similar cure in an elderly person. The difficulty of making choices led him to remark in subsequent correspondence, "I think only a fascist would suggest that older people should be denied treatment, but what I would suggest in more general terms is that factors such as proportion of man-years saved by treatment need to be taken into account when resources for health care are being allocated."

### Bone Marrow Transplantation

Bone marrow transplantation (BMT) is a new, expensive treatment for certain types of leukemia, one type of severe anemia, and several inherited disorders. It was first used to treat aplastic anemia, a disorder in which the bone marrow has been largely destroyed. Normally, marrow produces red and white blood cells and platelets. When the marrow is severely injured, the patient not only becomes anemic but becomes susceptible to severe hemorrhage and infection. Conventional treatment consists of giving transfusions and antibiotics in the hope that if the patient can be kept alive the bone marrow will recover spontaneously. Under this program fewer than one patient in four survives more than two years. BMT, which deals directly with the problem by providing new marrow cells, has boosted the survival rate to nearly half.[42]

BMT has also been used recently to treat certain forms of acute leukemia in which the prognosis for survival is poor with conventional therapy. Results are promising, though data from controlled clinical trials have not yet been reported.[43] BMT can also be used to treat certain rare inborn errors of metabolism and uncommon deficiencies of the body's immune system.

Patients with potentially treatable diseases can benefit from BMT only if two additional conditions are met. First, the patient must be young, usually under forty; older patients have an unacceptably high mortality rate. Second, a donor immunologically compatible with the potential recipient must be available. With few exceptions such donors are siblings.

### Method of Treatment

Bone marrow transplantation consists of the injection of bone marrow cells from a suitable donor into a vein of the patient. If the infused cells are not rejected, a normally functioning population of cells is reestablished in the marrow of the recipient. To accomplish this goal is, however, a complex and risky process because extreme measures must be taken to prevent rejection of the graft. The central requirement is that the patient's immune system be completely suppressed. This goal is accomplished by the administration of large doses of cytotoxic drugs, often combined with total body irradiation. Patients with leukemia are always subjected to total body irradiation in an attempt to eradicate all residual tumor cells and thus to prevent later recurrence. Graft rejection is rare in leukemia patients. By contrast, the graft is rejected in about 25 percent of cases of aplastic anemia, and in these patients transplantation is usually repeated.[44]

During the two- or three-week period before the graft begins to function, the patient is at considerable risk. The same measures that prevent the rejection of the bone marrow cells also suppress the patient's capacity to fight infection. Isolation facilities are used to minimize the chance of infection, and large doses of antibiotics are often required. During this same interval, red blood cell and platelet transfusions are administered to prevent fatal anemia.

Even if the transplant is successful, the patient still faces life-threatening problems. The transfused cells may react against the host's tissues, producing "graft-versus-host" disease. Moderate to severe graft-versus-host disease occurs in about 25 to 50 percent of patients and is fatal in one-quarter of the cases.[45] Severe pneumonia, from one or another DNA virus or bacterial infection, may also lead to death.

If all the problems are surmounted, the patient is usually cured and can return to a normal life. Some patients, however, may develop such long-term complications as chronic graft-versus-host disease. The total body irradiation may also cause cataracts or sterility or increase the incidence of a new cancer.

## Number of Patients

More than twenty BMT units in the United States carried out between 550 and 650 transplants in 1981. In the same year Britain had six transplant units able to do over 200 procedures annually, or a slightly larger capacity on a population-adjusted basis than in the United States. Most transplants in Britain are carried out on patients with acute leukemia. Even though Britain, relative to its population, has invested slightly more heavily in BMT than the United States has, the Department of Health and Social Security in 1981 reported a need for more units, primarily because all BMT facilities were in London and were operating close to capacity.[46]

## Cost

For many reasons bone marrow transplantation is very expensive. Costly isolation facilities, a staff of medical experts, and a high ratio of nurses to patients are all required. The unit must have access to an immunology laboratory and tissue-typing facilities. The long period of required hospitalization adds still another burden. It is thus not surprising that in 1978 the hospital charges at one leading U.S. center ranged from $35,000 to $66,000 per patient. BMT costs much less in Britain, $16,000 to $32,000 in 1980–81.[47] Total expenditure on bone marrow transplants in 1981 was thus about $30 million in the United States and $5 million in Britain. On a population-corrected basis, the British spent two-thirds as much as Americans.

## Total Parenteral Nutrition

Many illnesses severely impair a patient's ability to eat and thereby cause malnutrition. But until the 1970s it was not possible to provide full caloric and protein requirements except orally. Physicians could administer glucose intravenously but had no way of meeting the patient's total nutritional needs. It is now possible, however, to administer intravenously a solution containing not only enough calories but also enough amino acids to meet the body's total demands. Because this procedure, total parenteral nutrition (TPN), can prevent or correct malnutrition, it is an appealing therapeutic technique and has rapidly come into widespread use.

### Indications

TPN is effective in maintaining or restoring nutritional integrity, but this fact alone is an insufficient argument for its use. The procedure involves significant risks, which must be balanced against its benefits. For the procedure to be justified, one must show that treatment leads to improvement in one or another measure, such as mortality, morbidity, complications of the underlying disease, or length of hospital stay. Further, in evaluating the benefits of TPN, it is necessary to assess the results against alternative treatments, which are often easier to administer, safer, and less expensive. Patients, as mentioned earlier, can readily be given intravenous glucose to reduce the degree of tissue wasting, and many can also be fed by a tube inserted into the gastrointestinal tract. Most studies of the effectiveness of TPN have not included appropriate control groups. Enthusiastic support of the technique has more often been based on anecdotal experience than on randomized, prospective studies.[48]

TPN is demonstrably beneficial and better than alternative nutritional methods for only a small fraction of patients who receive it. It is often lifesaving for patients who have lost a large part of the small intestine, because they are usually incapable of taking any nourishment by mouth without developing severe diarrhea. It also appears to save the lives of premature infants with intractable diarrhea and to reduce mortality in patients with acute kidney failure. TPN may reduce both the mortality rate from surgery and the incidence of major postoperative complications among malnourished patients. Experts also believe that TPN helps cancer patients who have the potential of responding to chemotherapy but who cannot tolerate treatment because of malnutrition. But for most patients to whom TPN is administered—in particular, those with cancer (other than the kind described above), pancreatitis, inflammatory bowel disease, and burns—there is little evidence from controlled studies that TPN extends survival or reduces the frequency or severity of complications.[49]

A patient receiving TPN must be infused each day with one to four liters of nutrient-containing fluid. If the main source of calories is a concentrated glucose solution, the fluid must be administered through a long tube threaded into a large vein in the chest. The tube must end in a vessel that has a high blood flow because the elevated concentrations of glucose in the infusion damages small, superficial veins and soon makes them unusable. Peripheral veins can be used for TPN, however, if fat rather than glucose is the main caloric source; fat yields more than twice as many calories per gram as glucose and can be given in concentrations low enough to prevent unacceptable damage to veins in which blood flow is relatively low.

The central catheter has the advantage that it can often be left in place for weeks or months. But it also is a source of complications.[50] During insertion it may be misdirected, puncturing a lung or damaging other structures in the chest and causing hemorrhage. Blood clots may form where the catheter lies and require its immediate removal. Infection is the most serious complication. It can occur around the catheter, but meticulous care can keep the incidence to no more than a few percent of patients. Bacteria from an infection present elsewhere in the body may, however, seed the catheter through the blood stream. These complications, though sometimes serious, are rarely fatal. In any event, the medical decision on use of TPN must balance the risks from the potential complications, including some slight risk of death, against the potential benefits.

### Cost

Total parenteral nutrition is very expensive. Besides the solutions, there are large additional costs for pumps, tubing, catheters (including insertion), dressings, blood tests, and the time of nurses and pharmacists. Costs of inpatient TPN are estimated to be about $150 to $300 a day; the higher figures may overstate actual costs because they sometimes include charges for the patient's hospital room. Thus it appears that, on average, inpatient TPN, not counting room charges, costs at least $50,000 a year. The cost of home parenteral nutrition is much less, $20,000 to $30,000 a year.[51]

The cost of home parenteral nutrition in Britain is similar to that in the United States, ranging between $26,000 and $40,000 a year.[52] Data on the cost of inpatient TPN in Britain are not available; but even with the lower cost of personnel and routine supplies, the total cost is probably $30,000 to $40,000 a patient year.

Aggregate expenditures on total parenteral nutrition are much higher per capita in the United States than in Britain. Expenditures on TPN solutions in 1980 were $130 million in the United States but less than $8 million in Britain. Thus, on a population-corrected basis, Britain spent less than one-fourth as much as the United States.[53] To this figure must be added the costs of administering the solutions, with the result that total resource costs in the United States in 1980 were about $250 million a year and in Great Britain were about $15 million ($60 million, population corrected).[54]

### Reasons for Low British Expenditures

In theory, British physicians may provide as many patients as they wish with total parenteral nutrition. No special capital equipment is necessary. The physician simply orders the appropriate solutions from the pharmacy, inserts the needle or catheter, and directs nurses to supervise administration of the fluid. Nominally, there are no limits on the physician's ability to command pharmaceutical supplies. But in fact, financial stress results in sharp real restraints on the physician's nominal clinical freedom.

Experiences at two hospitals show how these limits evolve. In one large teaching hospital, we learned, the clinical interests of a consultant led to a steady growth in his expenditures on TPN. As other physicians began to prescribe it, rising costs pushed the hospital pharmacy over its budget. To make room for the TPN, the chief pharmacist cut back on maintenance, staff, and other services. Eventually the medical staff imposed a limit on TPN service. Even though the treatment often seemed effective, too much was being sacrificed. As one consultant put it, "Well, you know, you can say that all kinds of things are cost-effective. But why should preference be given to this? Why should large sums be spent on this kind of treatment when we can't have something else that would probably benefit a much larger group of patients?" In the end the staff decided to allow a maximum of six adult patients at a time to receive TPN.

A second large hospital responded to a similar rise in TPN expenditures by requiring the approval of a gastroenterologist before treatment could be started. Only the small intensive care unit was excepted. Consequently expenditure on solutions dropped by half within a year. In justifying the restrictions, the chief pharmacist stated, "We simply say, 'That is what we can do this week,' and that is a limitation that they must learn to live with."

Teaching hospitals face special pressures because they often are flooded with referrals from other institutions that do not have the service. Special budgetary provision is seldom made for the new procedure even though the hospital is providing a regional service.

Although Britain spends much less than the United States on TPN, its investment is substantial relative to its expenditures on other medical procedures about which there has been far more controversy. The British spend only $20 million on CT scanning and $30 million on coronary bypass grafts, for example. In the United States expenditures on TPN are roughly half as large as outlays on chronic dialysis and about the same as outlays on CT scanning.[55]

Despite such large expenditures, the very existence of TPN is unknown to most laymen and barely known to many policymakers concerned with costs. Because capital expenditures associated with TPN are negligible, the United States will have to use methods like those used in Britain that limit total hospital spending to curtail use of TPN.

## *chapter four* **Quality of Life**

People see doctors most often not because their lives are in danger but because they want help or reassurance about some problem that is making them physically or mentally uncomfortable. It is natural to suppose that if lifesaving medical care is constrained by a scarcity of resources, then care devoted to improving the quality of life will also be limited.

The story is a good deal more complicated than that, however. Surgery to replace arthritic hips can transform bedridden and pain-racked invalids into fully mobile and pain-free participants in normal life; the value of such care obviously compares favorably, for example, with the value of briefly extending the life of a semicomatose patient afflicted with a terminal disease. But care for chronic diseases, such as hernias or varicose veins, that cause protracted but not crippling discomfort may be regarded as dispensable.

Some diseases cause pain but do not render their victims incapable of living independent lives. Most people suffering from angina pectoris, for example, can care for themselves, and many can continue working if they are treated with appropriate drugs and moderate their activity. In a system strapped for resources, one would expect treatment of painful diseases that are neither disabling nor life threatening to be curtailed sharply relative to those that cause disability or require large custodial expenditures. Thus one might expect the British to curtail costly surgical treatment of angina to a far greater degree than they limit hip surgery. Such indeed is the case.

Because people with life-threatening diseases either receive treatment or die, whereas those with chronic diseases live on whether they are treated or not, the responses by patients and providers to limited resources differ in the two cases. For example, if resource limits necessitate some denial of care, perhaps those with chronic diseases can

57

be induced to get care from providers outside the budget limits and to pay for it themselves.


## Hip Replacement

One of the best known facts about the British health care system, both at home and abroad, is that the waiting lists for hip replacements are long and getting longer. In 1977 routine cases waited an average of thirteen to fourteen months and urgent cases an average of four months; barely concealed within these averages were extreme delays of up to five years, with even urgent cases waiting two or three years. Waiting lists grew 31 percent between 1977 and 1979.[1]


### *Waiting Lists and Waiting Times*

Large geographic variations in waiting lists and waiting times lie behind these averages. Consultants in poorly served regions claim that elective hip surgery inside the National Health Service has virtually ceased as acute traumatic cases absorb all available capacity. At the same time waiting lists are shorter and waiting times are reportedly briefer in the relatively well served London regions.[2] Only a few patients travel to take advantage of these differences, a finding that shows the importance attached to the provision of care near home and family.


### *The Procedure*

Because a badly deteriorated hip causes both pain and disability, doctors have long sought ways to alleviate these problems. The most radical approach involves replacing the joint completely. The hip is a relatively simple joint, an ordinary ball (at the end of the femur) and socket (in the pelvis), but because of the stress to which it is subject, an artificial joint must be strong and must also be able to resist corrosion by body fluids. Equally important, it must not cause inflammation.

Even after these problems were solved, hip replacement could not be done until a way was found to securely fasten the prosthesis to the remaining portion of the femur and to the pelvis. This problem proved the most difficult; not until the late 1960s was a new polymer plastic cement, polymethylmethacrylate, developed in Britain that seemed to give a bond with enough reliability and durability to make hip replacement feasible. The greatest danger in hip replacement is infection, the results of which can be catastrophic in that it may leave the patient much worse off than before. In addition, up to 5 percent of artificial hips annually loosen enough to cause symptoms. Hip replacements are far more successful for older patients, who can somewhat limit their activities, than for young patients, who usually subject the prosthesis to greater stress.[3] If the implanted joint loosens, the result may be discomfort, and repeat surgery is sometimes necessary. But the rate of loosening and the risk of infection and other complications are now low enough to make the procedure an excellent risk in patients with severe hip disease because the quality of the patient's life improves dramatically if the operation is successful.

Several kinds of hip procedures are now frequently performed, but total replacement of the hip, both the ball and socket, is the common procedure if the patient is elderly and if the disease is extensive. For a broken hip, also a common problem among the elderly, it is usually necessary to replace only the head and neck of the femur; in only a few instances is total hip replacement required.

### Frequency of Surgery

Data on the comparative frequency of hip replacement in Britain and the United States are hard to interpret because several different procedures are involved and reporting is incomplete. On a population-adjusted basis, the British do about three-quarters to four-fifths as many total hip replacements and nearly as much hip surgery of all kinds as Americans do (see the appendix). The very long waiting lists for hip replacement in Britain have arisen because the untreated patient does not get well and may live for years. Even a 25 percent shortfall in supply and only a four-year life expectancy among untreated patients will produce a waiting list equal to the number of patients who could be treated in one year.[4] In 1975 the waiting list for hip replacement contained about as many patients as could be treated in nine to twelve months.[5]

Waiting lists have persisted and grown in Britain despite an increase in resources devoted to orthopedic surgery. The number of consultants in trauma and orthopedic surgery increased 34 percent between 1969 and 1977. Between 1972 and 1978 there were a 3 percent increase in available beds, a 14 percent increase in consultants in orthopedic surgery, and a 15 percent increase in consultant anesthetists. Over the same interval there was only a 3 percent increase in the number of orthopedic outpatient visits. The number of orthopedic admissions rose 12 percent, from 423,200 in 1973 to 472,500 in 1977.[6]

This growth in resources for the discipline of orthopedic surgery made no dent in waiting lists for hip replacement, in part because the number of people in age brackets prone to hip problems increased rapidly: the population aged sixty-five and over rose by 12 percent between 1968 and 1978, and the number aged seventy-five and over increased by 20 percent.[7] Moreover, knowledge of hip replacement was spreading during the 1970s, and demand for the procedure was rising.

Opinions differ on which resource shortages are most to blame for the lengthy delays in treatment. British physicians and administrators frequently mention a shortage of beds, too few anesthetists, and a lack of operating room time.[8] Elective surgery always loses to emergency cases in the competition for resources. Emergency treatment of an elderly woman who has fallen and broken her hip will always take precedence over elective surgery to replace even a very painful arthritic hip.

Whatever the binding constraint may be, the foreign observer is prompted to wonder why the NHS allows the notorious and well-documented waiting lists for hip surgery to persist. Part of the reason is direct cost. To remove the backlog of hip surgery would cost roughly $200 million, about 1.2 percent of annual health expenditures. The fact is, however, that the very resources that would increase the capacity to provide hip replacements would be available for other uses as well. The hospital beds, the operating rooms, and hospital staff necessary for hip surgery can do other surgery and provide other nonsurgical care. The day-to-day allocation of health resources inside a hospital must fall to the doctors and nurses who decide which cases most need available time, beds, and supplies. Thus an administrative decision to add enough resources to eliminate even so highly visible a shortfall as the hip surgery backlog simply cannot be implemented unless hospital staff is persuaded that replacing more hips is more important than any other currently unmet demand. Without such a consensus, far more resources would be needed to end the queue for hip replacement than would be needed if they were allocated exclusively to hip surgery.

A large proportion of hip surgery, perhaps as much as 25 percent in some parts of Britain, according to informal estimates of DHSS officials and orthopedic consultants, is performed privately; that is, by doctors who see patients outside the NHS and who charge for their efforts on a fee-for-service basis. (The proportion is much lower in low-income areas, perhaps as low as 5 percent.) The operations may be performed in NHS pay beds or in private hospitals. Private insurance systems soften the financial blow for some private patients, but many pay the surgical fee and bed charges themselves.

The long waiting lists for hip surgery seem to invite manipulation by doctors who may spend part of their time treating patients privately on a fee-for-service basis. Where there are genuine limits on NHS care, the result would be quicker treatment for the patient and more income for the physician than if all were treated in the NHS. But some physicians might be tempted to maneuver patients into seeing them privately even if limitations on NHS care did not exist. A consultant could easily keep NHS beds fully occupied with other cases and tell candidates for hip surgery that a pay bed or a bed in a private hospital is available. Hip surgery is time consuming and exacting, and the surgeon could reason that several patients with other orthopedic problems could be treated in the lengthy period during which a patient must convalesce after hip surgery. There are no data on the extent of such practices. A group of orthopedic surgeons in one district general hospital gained some notoriety for allegedly doing a large part of their hip surgery on a private basis.[9] Some consultant physicians acknowledged hearing rumors that such practices occur, but most denied that they or any of their colleagues engaged in them.

But one British consultant made these comments on whether doctors manipulate waiting lists in order to encourage patients to see them privately: "It doesn't strike me as being improbable. I'm not talking about orthopedic surgeons, but I have heard gossip about this. I suspect that in certain places in this country patients may be encouraged to seek private treatment on a false basis, whereas they could get NHS treatment if they wished. But I think 95 percent of surgeons—and when I say surgeons, I should include physicians in all branches of private medicine—I think that 95 percent of them, if not more, operate on a very fair system. . . . But I've got pretty good evidence to indicate that in certain cities it does happen." And a colleague added, "I don't think any of us would deny it happens in this country. I think all of us would like to claim that we are at least as honest as most. We do our best, but it's a minority of black sheep."

Certainly the very possibility of waiting-list manipulation is one reason why some members of the Labour party strongly oppose the policy of letting physicians practice part-time for the NHS while also seeing patients privately.

From a broader standpoint, channeling patients into the private sector increases resources for health care without burdening government budgets. Few would condone such practices toward the acutely ill or the impecunious. But once a political decision has been made to curtail resources for hospital care, clearly some elective or nonurgent care that would be provided in an unconstrained system will not be given. In that event, providers might well want to focus on illnesses that cannot wait and patients who cannot pay.

### Coronary Artery Surgery

For nearly two hundred years doctors have understood that angina pectoris, the severe chest pain that typically radiates to the left arm and upward to the neck or jaw, is caused by a shortage of oxygen resulting from a diminished flow of blood to the heart muscle. For nearly that long they have been prescribing nitroglycerin and related drugs to relieve the pain. The pain arises because the arteries carrying blood to the heart muscle are narrowed by deposits that inhibit the flow of blood. Complete occlusion results in a heart attack and death of that portion of the heart denied oxygen. In recent years the number and variety of drugs available for treating angina have increased, relieving some patients not helped previously. These drugs sometimes provide so much relief that surgery can be postponed or even avoided.

### *Method of Treatment*

In recent decades surgical procedures have been developed for improving the flow of blood to the heart. Of these procedures coronary artery bypass surgery, first performed in 1974, is now used almost exclusively. Coronary artery bypass grafts became possible after the development of a machine that routes the patient's blood flow away from the heart, removes carbon dioxide from the blood, reoxygenates it, and returns it to the circulation. With the help of this machine, the heart can be stopped from pumping for long enough to permit surgical procedures on the heart itself.

Coronary artery surgery involves removing a vein from the patient's leg, or occasionally arm, and reattaching a segment of that vein both above and below the blocked section of the coronary artery; by this means blood can be detoured around that section. At first, the operation was highly risky. But over time the risk of death from surgery has declined, and operative mortality is now from 1 to 3 percent if the procedure is carried out by a team that does at least fifty operations a year.[10] The operation is never performed until detailed x-rays are taken of coronary arteries to determine the number and extent of blockages. This procedure, coronary arteriography or angiography, consists of inserting a tube into an artery through which radioopaque materials are injected into the coronary blood vessels so that they can be seen by x-rays.

One of the procedures that offer hope of reducing the need for coronary artery surgery is a variation of this diagnostic procedure. In addition to injecting contrast material, the physician introduces into the narrowed passage a catheter with a small balloon at its tip. Inflating the balloon usually crushes the obstructive lesion, thereby enlarging the opening and allowing an increased flow of blood.

## Cost

Coronary artery surgery, together with preparation and follow-up, cost $11,000 to $25,000 per patient in the United States in 1981. In 1982, 159,000 people underwent coronary artery surgery. The total cost was $2.5 billion to $3.0 billion in 1982, or roughly 1 percent of total U.S. health expenditures. It is estimated that the amount of coronary artery surgery could double.[11]

## Indications: Differences between Britain and the United States

Coronary artery surgery is clearly indicated for only a minority of patients: those who have disabling chest pain unresponsive to medical management and those whose prospects for survival can be substantially improved. Controversy surrounds the decision to operate on other patients, particularly because the procedure involves a small but significant risk and is very expensive. Surgery in roughly 10 percent of patients whose left main coronary artery is narrowed by more than 50 percent not only brings far more relief from pain than do drugs but also increases the chance of living at least five years by over 20 percentage points. In about 30 percent of all cases in which three or more arteries are affected, there is also some evidence that surgery prolongs life as well as reduces pain,[12] but British physicians in particular are skeptical about the studies on which this conclusion is based. In the remaining 60 percent of patients, the operation usually relieves pain more effectively than do available drugs, but it does not seem to affect life expectancy.

Thus statistics show that for approximately 70,000 of the 114,000 patients in the United States who underwent coronary artery surgery in 1979, the operation reduced cardiac pain but did not increase life expectancy. Of the remaining 44,000 patients, perhaps 5,000 who would have died without surgery were alive after five years.

Published data make abundantly clear that far less coronary artery surgery is done in Britain than in the United States. Whereas U.S. surgeons did about 490 coronary artery bypass operations per million population in 1979, British surgeons did about 55 per million in 1977.[13] Total expenditure in Britain was thus probably in the range of $20 million to $30 million.

What accounts for this very large difference? Five possible answers come to mind: differences in epidemiology, in available drugs for medical therapy, in physician and patient attitudes, in resources, and in the way physicians are paid. As becomes apparent, the first two answers may explain some, but not most, of the difference.

EPIDEMIOLOGY. More people die from coronary heart disease in the United States than in the United Kingdom. In 1969 the age-adjusted death rate from coronary heart disease was 290.8 per 100,000 in the United States, but this rate fell to 208.0 per 100,000 in 1982. In 1970, 189.9 people per 100,000 died from heart disease in the United Kingdom.[14] If the figures are carried over to coronary artery surgery, they would suggest that the eligible population is up to 50 percent larger in the United States than in Britain.

DRUGS. Two drugs, nifedipine and verapamil, unavailable until recently in the United States, are coming into increasing use. In some cases in which traditional drugs alone were ineffective, these agents are able to control pain.[15] During the period covered by our study, these and other agents were used aggressively and in various combinations in Britain. One British consulting cardiologist said that "this appreciably raised the threshold at which patients were referred for surgical treatment.'' But another distinguished cardiologist expressed doubt that differences in drug therapy account for any important difference in the indications for surgery in the two countries. Several experts in the United States believe that the recent introduction of nifedipine and verapamil has caused physicians to advise medical treatment for some patients who previously would have undergone a bypass, but they do not feel the effect has been large. Moreover, better drugs do not diminish the need for surgery in cases where surgery seems to improve life expectancy, that is, those with severe involvement of the left main artery or those suffering from three vessel disease. If the British operated only on these cases, 40 percent of the total, they would do 132 coronary artery operations per million population annually, more than twice their actual rate.[16] And to this group should, of course, be added the large number of patients whose pain is not controlled by drugs.

ATTITUDES. The medical indications for surgery are similar in the United States and Britain, but in describing when surgery is necessary, British and U.S. experts sound strikingly different. One example of British attitudes comes from an unsigned editorial in the *Lancet* in 1982:

It is still premature to offer coronary artery surgery to all patients with angina. Its use should be restricted to the proven indications of disabling chest pain, when full medical therapy has failed, and to the small group with extensive coronary artery disease and good left ventricular functions in whom mortality is reduced by surgery. Controlled clinical trials should be continued to define other areas of use.[17]

An example of U.S. attitudes comes from a report in the *New England Journal of Medicine*. The report outlines two extreme classes of cases where surgery clearly is and is not indicated. But it then goes on to say:

A very large percentage of patients fall between these extreme examples. In these patients, recommendations for medical or surgical therapy are based on two fundamental questions. The first question, often the most anxiety-provoking to the patient, relates to which course will provide the greatest protection from disabling myocardial infarction or death. The second question relates to which course will permit a satisfactory quality of life according to the patient's own standards. . . . The answer to the first is largely based on the physician's interpretation of a large volume of sometimes contradictory data of extraordinary complexity. The answer to the second is largely based on the individual response to medical therapy and to the patient's priorities.[18]

These two passages suggest that the two countries differ on how much the patient's attitudes and preferences count in the decision on whether to operate. The British editorial makes no reference to the preferences of the patient or to whether he willingly accepts the style of life and possible restriction of activity associated with medical treatment. A practicing general practitioner put the matter more concretely to us:

There are very few cases where coronary artery surgery is mandatory as an emergency. The typical case is treated to the full medically [in Britain]. Patients are asked to stop smoking. They are asked to lose weight. They are put on all of the different drugs. If they are still disabled then, or if it looks like it's a certain type of coronary artery disease, then one would refer them to a consultant a bit more quickly. And they would be seen by the consultant more promptly if I asked him to try to do it this week. Then the cardiologist decides what to do, whether or not to do arteriography, and if surgery is necessary it would usually be done in one to four months.

Another example of U.S. attitudes comes from a *Science* magazine article about the present consensus on coronary artery surgery:

It was also pointed out at the conference that many patients demand surgery rather than medical treatment. [T. Joseph] Reeves [director of the cardiovascular laboratory at St. Elizabeth's Hospital in Beaumont, Alabama] explained that male patients often "want to be seen as men, as husbands, as providers, and they are willing to risk their lives at the time of the operation so as not to change their life styles." [Vallee] Wilman [a cardiac surgeon at St. Louis University School of Medicine] mentioned still another reason why patients demand surgery. Their angina, he said, is a constant reminder that they are vulnerable to a heart attack or sudden death. "The patients want the consolation of having done everything possible. Surgery is at least a tangible assault on the process."[19]

A British internist reinforced these differences between U.S. and British attitudes in a letter:

I have been much involved with patients who have been investigated and subjected to surgery in the U.S.A., including some of the best medical centers there, and I have seen quite a lot of U.S. medicine first hand. What impresses me is that in comparison with the U.K. it seems very seldom that the U.S. physician ever states that there is no surgery that would help, no drug that is advantageous, and no further investigation that is required. There seems to be an irresistible urge always to *do something,* even though in many cases the doctor concerned must realize that there is no possibility of benefit.

Finally, another American cardiologist wrote us:

That there are fundamental differences in the personality structure of an Englishman versus an American seems to be well established throughout contemporary literature and the cartoons of our time. One has a "stiff upper lip," the other is flamboyant to the point of "wearing it on his sleeve." One, genteel and reserved, the other macho . . . the American demands surgery and . . . wants the consolation of having done everything possible. The Englishman tends to be more philosophical in approach and perhaps demands less.

British medical journals recognize that more coronary artery surgery should be done in Britain than present capacity permits. And there can be little doubt that the cardiologist is correct who stated that he believes "more CABG surgery would be carried out if the capacity for it increased significantly." But another British cardiologist noted, "It is absolutely true that in some parts of England resources are minimal so that surgical waiting lists are long and deaths occur during this period. However, in other areas there is in practice no limitation on resources and even here the rate of CABG surgery is lower than in the U.S."

RESOURCES AND METHODS OF PAYMENT. This whole picture must be set against the background of much lower rates of surgery of all kinds in Britain than in the United States.[20] Most U.S. surgeons are paid on a fee-for-service basis, whereas most British physicians are salaried employees of the NHS. In close calls the American physician will obviously have a greater incentive to carry out a bypass procedure than his British counterpart. As one American cardiologist put it: "The entrepreneurial aspect of surgery in this country makes it imperative for surgeons to pursue the recruitment of patients aggressively. There is not only the major income motivation, but also the need to meet all sorts of state standards in terms of the number of cases done per year, solely to justify a cardiac surgical unit's existence (greater than 250 in many states)." Experts tell us that, probably as a result of these considerations, the criteria for coronary artery surgery vary widely among U.S. hospitals, with considerable homogeneity among the large centers but much variation elsewhere.

Finally, U.S. and British resources are vastly different. To match American rates of coronary artery surgery would cost the British about $200 million, or about 1 percent of their health budget. This amount, as mentioned earlier, is close to the annual increment in total British health expenditures in recent years.

*chapter five* **More Reliable Diagnoses**

Patients like to think that physicians diagnose ill-nesses with certainty and then prescribe the uniquely best treatment to effect a cure. Indeed, this faith may play a constructive therapeutic role, because tension from doubt and uncertainty can cause patients to deviate from prescribed regimens and can directly obstruct recovery.

The truth, however, is quite different. As some patients and all doctors realize, physicians are often unsure about the precise cause of various signs and symptoms. More information frequently leads to certainty about the diagnosis and increased confidence in choosing a course of treatment. Indeed, the science of getting the best information and using it logically is the essence of good medicine.[1]

Physicians have many techniques for obtaining information. Tests for determining the concentration of dozens of constituents of blood, urine, sputum, and other body components have long been available, and new techniques for measuring the previously unmeasurable are constantly appearing. In a like manner, traditional x-ray examinations of body structure are being augmented or replaced by procedures that use sound, radioisotopes, nuclear magnetic resonance, fiberoptics, and x-rays linked to computers. These instruments dramatically improve information and diagnoses in some cases. But many of these procedures are very costly, and the value of the information is often small. Are the improvements in information worth the cost?

One would expect that answers to this question would depend on the availability of resources. Where resources are quite limited, we antici-pate increased caution and skepticism about making sizable expenditures to improve diagnostic procedures. Before budget-constrained decision-makers make large investments in new techniques, they would have reason to insist on being shown the value of the information to be gained.

Comparison of investments in Britain and the United States in two forms of diagnostic equipment supports those expectations. British scientists pioneered the development of computed tomographic (CT) scanning, a technique that provides detailed information about body structures in a noninvasive fashion. Nevertheless, Britain has been slow to invest in such scanners. At the same time, the British have economized on conventional x-rays by keeping old machines in service longer than is common in the United States, performing fewer examinations and using less film per patient.

The crucial question is whether these economies have caused large sacrifices in the quality of medical care. This question is crucial because many health economists and planners, and some physicians, hold that the United States has overinvested in CT scanners and question whether many of the x-rays performed are necessary.

## CT Scanners

Computed tomography is a fairly new addition to the range of techniques capable of producing pictures of the internal structure of the human body in a physically noninvasive way. A CT scanner is an x-ray machine linked to a computer. The computer processes the information from multiple x-ray beams focused on the patient from different angles and produces a cross-sectional picture at any site along the length of the body. In this way sequential "slices" of brain, liver, spine, and other tissues can be visualized in detail, all without greater risk or pain to the patient than that produced by ordinary x-rays. Unlike x-rays, which poorly differentiate among various kinds of soft tissues, the CT scanner distinguishes, for example, brain tissue from tumor or a liver abscess from normal liver substance. The CT scanner also makes it possible to identify the size of such abnormalities and to pinpoint their location.

Other techniques for producing even more accurate images or different kinds of information are now under development.[2]

The rate of technical advance in the CT scanner is impressive. The first scans took five minutes or longer per exposure, and five minutes of computer time to analyze the result; because movement of the torso associated with breathing blurred the pictures, scanners initially were designed for the head only. But new scanners can now be used on any part of the body because exposures on them take three seconds or less.

As exposure time has shrunk, picture quality has improved, increasing steadily the number of situations in which CT scans can provide useful information. The issue now is how useful information must be to justify the average charge of roughly $300 per scan. CT scans have largely or totally replaced a number of diagnostic procedures that are less accurate, create discomfort for the patient, carry significant risks, or cost more than CT scans.[3]

### Cost

A new top-of-the-line CT scanner costs about $700,000 (though stripped-down and reconditioned models can be had for much less, some for under $100,000). Annual running costs have been estimated at roughly $300,000 in the United States and are not proportionately less for less expensive machines. Adding depreciation, interest, and running costs produces estimates of the total annual cost of operating a body scanner as high as $420,000, and even if the unit employs a second-hand machine, the cost may be close to half as much.[4]

The cost per scan depends on how much the machine is used, because most of the costs do not vary with the volume of examinations. In 1976 the average cost per scan, including professional fees, ran about $340 if the machine was used for 1,300 scans a year and about $220 if the machine was used for 2,600 scans a year.

As with many other services provided by expensive equipment, the average cost of a CT scan (total cost divided by number of scans) differs greatly from the marginal cost of one more scan. To do any scans at all, one must buy a machine and hire and train the staff to operate it. Once these costly steps are taken, the incremental expense of doing one more scan is small if the machine is uncongested. At some point, as use increases, one must either hire more staff to run a night shift (often impossible because of the internal rhythm of a hospital) or buy and staff another machine. The incremental, or marginal, cost for each additional scan was about $25 in 1976.[5] These costs were probably about 30 percent higher in 1982. Since prices of scanners have risen more slowly than prices in general, capital costs now constitute a smaller fraction of total costs than in the past. The cost per scan also depends on the time required to perform it, some scans requiring more than twice as long as others.[6]

CT scans seem to cost less in Britain than in the United States—at least the British think they do. The British assume that the useful life of a machine is longer than Americans assume, and labor costs are markedly less in Britain than in the United States, most notably for professional fees. When all factors are taken into account (except interest costs), the British perceive the cost of a scan to be about $140, the Americans about $280.[7] All told, the British spent about $10 million on CT scanning in 1979 and would have to quintuple spending to achieve U.S. levels of service.

### Number of Scanners and Scans

With adjustment for population, the United States has about three times as many head scanners and ten times as many body scanners as Britain does.[8] But Japan has as many machines as the United States for a population half as large, and a recent NIH consensus panel concluded that the United States has too few machines.[9] The United States could easily make effective use of two to three times as many as it does. The greater difference between Britain and the United States in the relative numbers of body and head scanners reflects the fact that during the early period when only head scanners were available, real health expenditures were rising in Britain. By the time that body scanners became the preferred machine because of their greater versatility, resources in Britain were highly constrained.

Data on use are less reliable than those on numbers of scanners. On the basis of published estimates, the United States does 3.4 more scans per capita on head scanners than do the British, ten times more scans on body scanners, and roughly five times more scans in all.[10]

### Charity

Although the differences between scanning capacity in the United States and Britain are great, they would be even larger were it not for the important role played by private charity in Britain. Of thirty-three body scanners in place or on order in late 1980, sixteen were paid for fully or partially by donated funds or from hospital endowments.[11] Three or four of the thirty-three head scanners are reported to have been donated. Operating expenses are usually not covered by donations but must be met by the health authorities from their own funds.

*Looking Ahead*

The CT scanner represents a growing class of diagnostic procedures dependent on costly equipment that must be run at high volume to keep average costs down. For several good reasons every hospital would like to have access to such equipment. The CT scanner is a convenient, noninvasive instrument that can be used to diagnose a wide variety of diseases, to confirm diagnoses and aid in the treatment of others. Although it is possible to transport patients from one hospital to another, it is sometimes dangerous and almost always inconvenient and time consuming to do so. One radiologist expressed to us the opinion that any hospital with 200 or more beds and a diverse caseload could justify having a CT scanner; on this criterion, the United States would eventually have more than 3,000 scanners. The position of the NIH consensus panel is consistent with this view. Even smaller hospitals could make part-time use of portable scanners mounted on trucks. According to a noted British radiologist, the British aim eventually to have 100 scanners in England and Wales. If the goals of both countries are reached, the United States would continue to have about six times the scanner capability of England and Wales on a population-adjusted basis.

In Britain the purchase of CT scanners must compete within the total health budget for available funds. Although it would cost Britain only $80 million, or less than 1 percent of hospital expenditures, to achieve the same availability and use of CT scanners as in the United States, the British authorities have elected not to spend that money. Almost certainly, the financial saving has had as its price a substantial reduction in the quality of care.

## Diagnostic X-Rays

One might suppose that budget limits would not affect so basic a service as diagnostic x-rays to the same extent as they curtail high-technology medicine. But this supposition would be wrong. In Britain the effects of budget limits are apparent in purchases of x-ray equipment, in the way the equipment is staffed, in the number of patients undergoing x-ray examinations, and in the amount of film used for each patient. In each aspect, economies are evident relative to U.S. practice. The cumulative effect is a manyfold difference in expenditures.

The United States performs nearly two times more x-ray examinations per capita and uses four times as much film as does Britain.[12] It appears, therefore, that the average British citizen is about half as likely to be x-rayed as the average American, and when he is x-rayed about half as much film is likely to be used. The British would have to spend an additional $500 million, more than 2 percent of annual health expenditures, to match U.S. levels of x-ray use.

This difference exists partly because British GPs seldom have x-ray machines in their offices, whereas many American physicians do. More important is the fact that NHS radiology departments are understaffed, predominantly lacking in radiologists rather than technicians. Workloads are heavy, and a good percentage of routine films are not seen by radiologists but by more junior staff, with loose supervision. The problem appears to be a shortage of trained physicians rather than of staff positions. One radiologist we interviewed estimated that about forty to fifty staff positions are currently unfilled nationwide; another estimated the number to be as high as seventy-five to a hundred. Furthermore, two DHSS officials estimate that radiological services in the National Health Service lack 200 to 300 full-time-equivalent radiologists.[13]

There are several probable reasons for the shortage of radiologists in Britain: (1) training programs are few and limited in size, (2) many radiologists emigrate, (3) incomes are lower than in other specialties because opportunities for private practice are few, and (4) the DHSS deliberately wants to hold down the number of radiologists to curtail unnecessary or marginally beneficial x-rays. In 1978 there were 10,820 radiologists (including residents) in the United States, or 5 radiologists per 100,000 population, compared with 2.4 consultants, senior registrars, and registrars in radiology departments in NHS hospitals in England and Wales per 100,000 population, a ratio of more than 2 to 1.[14] Even if the 300 British radiologists were added to the group, there would still be only slightly more than half as many radiologists per capita in Britain as in the United States.

Although the number and extent of x-ray examinations is constrained by the shortage of radiologists, we have no evidence that it is further constrained by a shortage of capital equipment. But the quality of the equipment, and therefore of the radiologic studies, is, on average, far lower in Britain than in the United States. We base this assertion on the fact that the British per capita expenditure on diagnostic x-ray machines is only one-fourth that of the United States.[15] The consequence, inevitably, is that the equipment must be less sophisticated and must be kept in service far longer than is common here. Most tellingly, expenditures on x-ray services in the United States totaled $27.66 per capita in 1977, compared with $3.40 in the National Health Service.[16] Private sector outlays add a small amount to the British figure, but even after that addition, U.S. x-ray outlays are roughly seven times those of Britain.

The effect on health care is hard to assess. We were told that in many British hospitals x-rays are difficult or impossible to get at night or on weekends except in emergencies and that such time-consuming tests as barium examinations of the gastrointestinal tract have long waiting lists. In contrast, U.S. patients may undergo too many x-rays from physicians anxious to obtain the slight amount of additional information that another study will provide but unheedful of the extra cost and of the long-run risks that additional exposure to x-rays entail.[17] The tendency to order too many x-rays may also be exacerbated by fear of malpractice suits.

On balance, it appears that British staffs are large enough to deal with the cases in which the payoff from an x-ray is high. But it is doubtful that the British can provide information as accurately or quickly as Americans or deal with cases in which a study has a relatively low expected value. There are many patients for whom the payoff from an additional x-ray is small—the confirmation of a diagnosis or the elimination of a small possibility—and in those cases the British do not perform x-rays or, if they do, take fewer films. The critical question concerns the size of potential benefits sacrificed when budget limits preclude x-rays in marginal situations. If, as seems likely, this curve declines rapidly, then economies in a routine procedure such as x-rays are a rational response to limited resources.

## Summary

The British, on a per capita basis, buy less than Americans of many of the technological procedures discussed in this part of the book. They provide the same volume of care only for radiotherapy, bone marrow transplantation, and the treatment of hemophilia. At the other end of the spectrum lies coronary artery surgery; the British do only 10 percent as many procedures per capita as Americans. In a few instances, such as cancer chemotherapy, differences in clinical judgment may possibly explain all the differences between the number of patients cared for in

**Table 5-1. Approximate Annual Cost of Increasing Selected Services in Britain to U.S. Levels, 1979, 1980, or 1981**

Millions of dollars

| Service | Added cost for full service |
|---|---|
| Bone marrow transplantation | 0 |
| Cancer chemotherapy | 40 |
| CT scanners | 80 |
| Coronary artery surgery | 175 |
| Diagnostic x-rays | 500 |
| Hemodialysis | 140 |
| Hemophilia | 0 |
| Hip replacement | 50 |
| Radiotherapy | 0 |
| Total parenteral nutrition | 45 |
| Subtotal | 1,030 |
| Intensive care beds | 1,365 |
| Total | 2,395 |
| Total hospital expenditures in 1980 | 12,960 |

Sources: Authors' estimates based on data in part 2 and the appendix. The estimates are based on British service costs, which in many cases are well below U.S. costs. Because differences between British service levels and full care are approximations, as explained in part 2, the estimates are subject to some uncertainty.

Britain and in the United States. But in the case of such procedures as coronary artery surgery and CT scans, resource limits have led the British to sacrifice some medically beneficial information or treatment. The political process implicitly concluded that the benefits were worth less than the value of alternative objects of public expenditure.

The financial stakes are large, as shown in table 5-1, which reports rough estimates of the annual costs the British would have to incur to bring eleven services up to U.S. levels. At one extreme, the British provide full treatment of hemophilia, bone marrow transplantation, and radiotherapy, though even for the last procedure the British have achieved some economies in staffing that may result in some loss of quality. In all other areas, service levels are well below those that would be necessary to treat all patients who could benefit at quality levels similar to those in the United States.

The British would have had to spend an additional $1.030 billion around 1980 to have provided full care, and a total of $2.395 billion if intensive care is included. These amounts may seem modest by American standards or compared with the range of improvements that could be achieved. But it represents roughly an 8 percent increase over British hospital expenditures in 1980, 18 percent if intensive care is included. In a system that has managed annual growth in real outlays of only 1.5 percent a year, however, such increases would require a major change in the priority attached to health care. It is precisely such a change that neither Labour nor Conservative governments since 1975 have been prepared to make.

The most striking aspect of these comparisons is that the pattern of rationing evident in Britain is so uneven: Britain provides some services in negligible quantities and some at nearly the same levels as found in the much less constrained U.S. system.

*part three* **Coping with Scarcity**

*chapter six* **Rationing and Efficiency**

Every nation must decide how much to spend on medical care and which services to buy. The decision on how much to spend expresses a judgment about the value of medical services relative to that of other consumption and investment. Whether Britain or the United States spends more or less than it "should" is an issue that we are unqualified to resolve. Decisions on medical care vary from country to country because of differences in incomes, prices, and tastes. For example, per capita medical care expenditure and the proportion of national income devoted to medical care rise more than proportionately with per capita income.[1] Thus the United States spends a larger share of its national income on health care than does Britain in part because it is richer than Britain. And because doctors' salaries are lower relative to average wages in Britain than in the United States, a given expenditure buys more health care in Britain than in the United States.

Whatever the amount spent on medical care, one must also consider the efficiency with which medical expenditures are allocated. Given that Britain spends less on medical care than the United States, does it get as much medical benefit as possible from the expenditures it makes? And given that Britain provides far less of some forms of care than the United States, but nearly as much of other forms, do such differences make medical sense?

Addressing these questions requires an explicit understanding of efficiency. Medical resources are efficiently used when a given total expenditure cannot be reallocated to alternative kinds of care to achieve an improved medical outcome. In the first section we apply the concept of efficiency to medical care to explain why a nation bent on curtailing the growth of expenditures might cut different services by different amounts. Then we estimate how much of the difference between British expenditures and U.S. expenditures stems from the technologies we have described. In chapter 7 we try to evaluate the British decisions about which services to curtail, using this standard of efficiency and our judgments of medical effectiveness and social priorities.

### Medical Efficiency

The benefits produced by expenditures on medical care are many and complex. Medical ethics prohibit courses of action expected to produce harmful outcomes but require doctors to recommend any action, however costly, that is expected, on balance, to help the patient. Not all actions produce the desired benefits, and some may cause harm; but the combination of possible outcomes, appropriately weighted for their probability, must be of benefit to the patient to make a course of action ethically acceptable. Sometimes people may not agree about how beneficial a certain outcome will be or even whether it will be beneficial or harmful. Thus extending the life of a pain-ridden, terminally ill patient may be viewed differently by the physician, the patient, and the patient's family. Because medical care is not an exact science, physicians continue to disagree about the likelihood of various outcomes of a course of action with a particular patient; and because tastes, values, and circumstances vary, people will weigh differently the desirability of a given set of outcomes.

Despite these complications, it is possible to speak meaningfully of a benefit curve for medical procedures. Imagine that a calculation is done showing the "expected social value" per dollar of expenditure on different forms of health care provided to each patient. A physician undertakes a medical procedure because it has some probability of improving the clinical outcome for a patient. The benefit from the procedure consists of the hoped-for clinical gain and the value placed on the range of possible outcomes by the patient, his family, and sometimes society at large. Expected social value is the product of the probability and the value placed on the clinical benefit.

Expressing benefits per dollar of expenditure helps one to compare the benefits of, say, routine x-rays with those of coronary artery surgery. It does not mean that one must place a money value on the benefits of health care. It does mean that, at least subjectively, one must be willing to compare the value of diverse services producing very different effects.

Imagine that these expected values are listed from largest to smallest.

A curve can be drawn to show how the expected value of the last dollar of care declines as the number of people served and the level of service per person increases. The expected clinical gains from treatment cannot, however, be measured precisely. For example, the expected clinical gain from coronary artery surgery, a CT scan, or treatment for cancer on a linear accelerator involves much uncertainty, reflected in statements on the probability of given physical or emotional results. Furthermore, the valuation of benefits may depend on nonmedical factors, such as the patient's age, his underlying health or family responsibilities, and perhaps his social position. For some dread diseases, such as cancer, society may invest heavily because it derives comfort from the knowledge that everything possible is being done, even when the prospects for recovery or improvement are slight.

Figure 6-1 illustrates benefit curves with different shapes.* Some therapies—splinting broken bones or liver transplants, for example—produce large benefits for a clearly defined population, but none for anyone else (procedure A). Other therapies—CT scans, for example—produce large benefits for a few people and small benefits for a very large population (procedure B). Still other therapies may produce gradually decreasing benefits as expenditures on them increase (procedure C).

If all medically beneficial care were provided and the benefit curves were as drawn in the figure, most money would be expended on hypothetical procedure B, least on hypothetical procedure A. No ethical problem would arise for providers because all procedures yielding any expected benefits would be offered regardless of cost. We refer to this level of service as full care.

If some beneficial care is not provided—for example, because the cost is disproportionate to the resulting benefits—one must decide what care for which specific patients will not produce benefits as great as the cost. Some people believe that when health care is involved, any reference to cost is repugnant, even immoral. It is doubtful that such a belief was ever defensible. But the rising cost of medical care, in our opinion, has made that belief untenable, because some of the increasing quantity of resources spent on medical care might yield a larger return if applied to other uses. As soon as one determines in some way, other

---

* The precise shape of the curves in figure 6-1 has no empirical basis, although we are persuaded that, in general, the contrasting shapes represent the benefits of various services. "Units of care" are defined as the quantity of a service that can be purchased for $1.00.

**Figure 6-1. Benefit Curves for Three Hypothetical Medical Procedures**

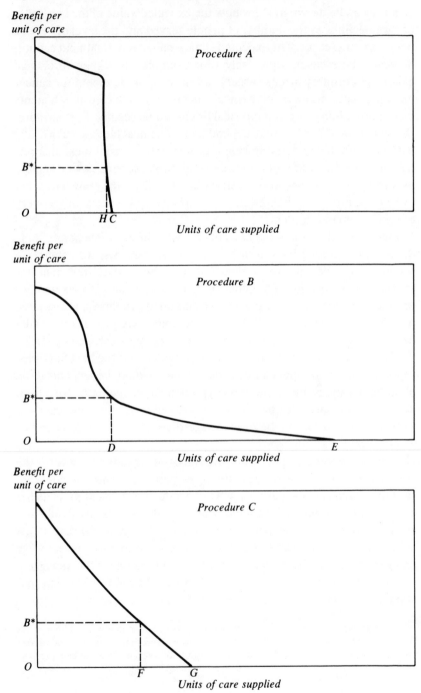

than by caprice or lottery, not to provide all care that is expected to yield benefits, the value of care is being weighed against its costs, explicitly or implicitly. Care actually given is implicitly judged to be worth more than it costs; care not given is worth less.

If only those procedures that produce benefits greater than some arbitrary level (shown as $B^*$ in figure 6-1) were provided, the quantity spent on each of the hypothetical procedures would decline, but by widely different proportions.* The amount spent on procedure A, for example, would decline negligibly (from $OC$ to $OH$), whereas that on procedure B would decline greatly (from $OE$ to $OD$). Expenditures on procedure C would be affected moderately (from $OG$ to $OF$).

Whatever the overall level of expenditure, however, two central points emerge. First, the efficient use of resources in medical care (or in any other field) requires that the benefit from the last dollar spent in any activity be no lower than the benefit obtainable from spending an additional dollar on some other procedure or for some other patient. As Alan Williams put it, "Only when we can be satisfied that the most valuable thing that we are not doing is less valuable than the least valuable thing that we are doing, can we be sure that we are being efficient in the pursuit of welfare."[2] Second, a decision not to provide full care but to offer only care that yields benefits greater than some minimum (such as $B^*$ in figure 6-1) will have very different quantitative implications for different procedures. For analogous reasons, some reductions in quality may be required for efficiency.

Benefit curves apply, of course, not just to medical care but to all useful goods and services. Economists call them demand curves, the schedule of values that consumers attach to successive units of a commodity. People are thought to buy goods up to the point where the value of one more unit is less than the price they must pay for it. Because people usually ignore benefits or costs that accrue to people other than the buyer, a person's demand curve is usually taken to represent the total benefits a commodity provides to him.

---

* The text ignores a complication of great practical importance. What constitutes the "cost" of a procedure is often far from clear. Procedures that require costly capital equipment, for example, may require a large expenditure to provide the service in the first instance. But additional patients can be served at modest cost until the capacity of the machine is reached or until the machine has to be run for more than one normal work shift. In such situations the average cost of a procedure is far above the marginal cost of serving one more person, at least until the machine becomes congested. As shown in chapter 5, this cost pattern applies to CT scanners.

The demand for medical care, however, is not a simple expression of the value patients place on it. Patients often have little understanding of the benefits that a given type of care can be expected to yield. Even if patients have some idea, private insurance or public programs relieve them of most incentives to weigh benefits and costs. Similarly doctors, because of both professional ethics and the threat of malpractice suits, have little incentive to do so either. For these reasons, a person's demand curve for medical care is not a social benefit curve in the same sense that the demand curves for restaurant meals and movie admissions are.

### Health Expenditures in the United States and Britain

All health systems ration care to some degree, but the severity of budget limits in Britain makes the choices about what services *not* to provide more agonizing than any such choices in the United States or in most other developed countries. As noted earlier, the difference in per capita health expenditures is a key measure of the severity of British constraints: expenditures in Britain are just over one-third of those in the United States (table 6-1).

For many reasons, however, that difference is a misleading guide to the severity of budgetary limits on hospital care. First, the incidence of illnesses differs markedly from country to country. Death from heart disease, for example, has been more common in the United States than in Britain. In 1969, 290.8 people per 100,000 population died from heart disease in the United States. By 1982, this rate had fallen to 208.0 per 100,000. In 1970, 189.9 people per 100,000 died from heart disease in Britain. By contrast, death from cancer occurs less frequently in the United States than in Britain. Second, health expenditures tend to rise with the average age of the population, and the British population is somewhat older than that of the United States; in 1980, 14.6 percent of the British population was sixty-five or older, compared with 11.3 percent of the U.S. population. Although these two factors may be significant, we lack enough reliable data to take them into account.[3]

In table 6-1, however, we make other adjustments to hospital expenditures. First, we exclude expenditures that do not directly affect patient care in the short run (line 2). Administrative costs are real, but because the organization of health care in Britain is very different from that in the United States and because administrative expenditures affect

**Table 6-1. Per Capita Health Expenditures in the United States and Britain, 1978**
Dollars per capita

| Item | United States | Britain |
|---|---|---|
| 1. Total health expenditures | 862.50 | 308.40 |
| 2. Less expenditures on administration, research, construction, and depreciation | 780.74 | 286.90 |
| 3. Less pay advantage in the United States of doctors and other health personnel | 602.90 | 286.90 |
| 4. Less dental services, outpatient drugs, eyeglasses, nursing homes, government public health, and other nonhospital services: | | |
|     Equals hospital expenditures | 327.33 | 173.96 |
| 5. Difference between per capita hospital expenditures in the United States and Britain | 153.37 | |

Source: Authors' estimates based on data reported in Jeremy W. Hurst, "Aggregate Comparison of the Performance of the American and British Health Sectors" (London: Department of Health and Social Security, n.d.), table C-1.

patient care only indirectly, we deduct them. Because the effects of research on patient care are deferred and indirect, we also exclude these expenditures. And because of differences in accounting, we deduct outlays on new construction and depreciation.

Second, we make a crude adjustment for the fact that U.S. doctors are better paid relative to average per capita income than are their British counterparts (line 3). These statistics are not adjusted for possible differences in productivity. Doctors and other health personnel are paid more in the United States than in Britain. Part of this difference reflects the generally higher per capita income in the United States than in Britain; part reflects an extra pay advantage of medical personnel over other workers in the United States. If medical workers are equally productive in the two countries, these differences in pay will not represent differences in services. For many reasons the productivity of health personnel may differ in the United States and Britain, despite the similarity of standards of health care and methods of training. Table 6-1 assumes that the average productivity of physicians and other health personnel in Britain and the United States is the same.*

---

* This assumption is almost certainly false, but we make it because the polar opposite assumption—that all of the differential reflects differences in the productivity of health personnel—strikes us as even farther from the truth, and because we have no accurate way of measuring what intermediate position the truth is likely to occupy.

The assumption that differences in pay reflect no differences in productivity would hold true only if the amount of medical equipment and other facilities per physician and

Third, in table 6-1 we exclude health expenditures other than those made for hospital based medical services, such as dental care, eyeglasses, outpatient drugs, and nursing home care (line 4).*

After incorporating the relevant adjustments, we find that per capita expenditures on hospital care in Britain were 53 percent of those in the United States.**

Much of the $153.57 difference between British and U.S. expenditures on health care antedates the development of most of the procedures that we have studied. As early as 1960 the British spent $67.02 (in 1978 prices)

---

other health workers were the same in the United States and Britain or if such capital equipment had no effect on medical productivity. The United States employs slightly more physicians and many more other medical personnel than Britain does; the United States, therefore, has more "standard health workers" than Britain, a standard health worker being an appropriately weighted average of doctors and other health personnel. The United States also has more medical capital than Britain. We lack data to calculate the difference in the value of the capital stocks of Britain and the United States and to measure how many standard health workers each country has. Consequently, we are unable to estimate the capital per standard health worker in the two countries. Nonetheless, all available data indicate that U.S. health care workers have more capital than their British counterparts. If this supposition is correct, then capital should increase the productivity of American physicians and other medical workers.

Even if the amount of capital per worker were the same, however, productivity might differ, because of differences in education, training, or other factors. We have not tried to measure the effects that any such influences might have.

* The deduction of nursing home care overstates British expenditures relative to those in the United States because British statistics do not list nursing home expenditures separately. Some British hospitals provide care for elderly patients that might be provided in the United States in skilled or intermediate nursing facilities. We are unable to estimate the size of those expenditures. To facilitate comparison, it is useful to note that per capita nursing home expenditure in the United States in 1978 was $68. Jeremy W. Hurst, "Aggregate Comparison of the Performance of the American and British Health Sectors" (London: Department of Health and Social Security, n.d.), table C-1.

** Unfortunately, comparisons of expenditures among countries based on exchange rates are notoriously unreliable when the commodities involved are not traded internationally. Medical expenditures suffer from this potential problem because they consist mostly of the direct services of physicians and other health care workers. We have tried, crudely, to adjust for this problem by considering the differences between the relative pay of medical workers in the two countries. But this approach is conceptually unsatisfactory for reasons indicated in the note on page 85. Drugs and much equipment are internationally traded; but even for such commodities sizable differences in prices may persist. The large difference between the price of factor VIII concentrate in the United States and that in Britain, cited in chapter 3, is an example.

Despite the conceptual shortcomings of our calculations, we believe that the difference between per capita hospital expenditures in Britain and the United States, shown in table 6-1, reasonably approximates the difference in resources used for hospital services in the two countries.

**Table 6-2. Sources of the Difference between Per Capita Hospital Expenditures in Britain and the United States, Late 1970s**

| Item | Amount (dollars) | Percent of increment in difference |
|---|---|---|
| Excess of U.S. over British per capita expenditures on hospital care, 1978 | 153.57 | ... |
| Less excess of U.S. over British per capita expenditures on hospital care, 1960 | 67.02 | ... |
| Increment in difference, 1960–78 | 86.55 | 100 |
| Difference attributable to ten procedures described in part 2 | 17.87 | 21 |
| Dialysis | 2.51 | ... |
| Treatment of hemophilia | 0 | ... |
| Therapeutic radiology | 0 | ... |
| Cancer chemotherapy | 0.71 | ... |
| Bone marrow transplantations | 0 | ... |
| Total parenteral nutrition | 0.27 | ... |
| Hip replacement | 0.89 | ... |
| Coronary artery surgery | 3.13 | ... |
| Computed tomography (CT) | 1.43 | ... |
| Diagnostic radiology | 8.93 | ... |
| Difference attributable to greater availability of intensive care in the United States than in Britain | 24.38 | 28 |
| Other causes of difference | 44.30 | 51 |

Source: Authors' calculations based on data in part 2.

less than the United States on health care, compared with $153.37 less in 1978 (table 6-2).[4] The procedures that we have examined account for nearly half of the $86.55 increase in the difference between outlays in the two countries that has arisen since 1960.

The extra costs the British would incur if they provided each of the services we have examined to all patients who would benefit from them is shown in table 6-2. (Whether the British decision not to make these expenditures has been well considered is an important question examined in the next chapter.) The table also includes a crude estimate of what it would cost the British to increase the proportion of intensive care beds to the U.S. level. Some considerable further part of this difference is undoubtedly caused by limits on the resources applied to technologies other than those that we studied. A few examples are enough to effectively illustrate this point. Over the last decade large expenditures have been made in this country on fetal monitoring, ultrasound, nuclear medicine, angiography, cardiac catheterization, and immunology labo-

ratories. Investment in smaller high-technology activities, such as am-
niocentesis and balloon dilation of narrowed blood vessels, has also
proceeded apace. In many of these specialized areas, highly sophisticated equipment and computers have replaced simpler and less expensive devices. Although we made no direct study of these procedures,
our assessment suggests that the British spend far less on these activities
than do Americans. Nor did we take into account the far more extensive
and expensive use of clinical tests in the United States and the greater
shift from wards to private rooms in U.S. hospitals.

These comparisons enable one to reject the hypothesis that budget
limits operate solely on high technologies that must compete with
established services for resources. But they establish that newly developed treatments account for most of the increment in the difference
between per capita hospital expenditures in Britain and the United
States. If tight budget limits endure for as long as they have in Britain,
they cause significant economies in the provision of a broad range of
medical services, though the effects on new technologies are disproportionate. And as science continues to spawn new and costly diagnostic
and therapeutic procedures, the maintenance of budget limits in Britain
promises ever more wrenching choices about delays in the introduction
of new techniques and the curtailment of old ones. The difference
between the United States and Britain in the provision of chronic dialysis,
coronary artery surgery, TPN, and intensive care is proportionally far
greater than the difference between total spending in the two countries
on health care in general or on hospital care. We now turn to the question
whether the paucity of these services in Britain represents a medically
rational response to budget limits.

*chapter seven* **Efficiency and Inefficiency**
**in British Health Care**

Efficiency in use of medical resources means that the last dollar spent on any particular type of care purchases medical benefit worth no less than the last dollar spent for any other type of care. This is just another way of saying that if resource allocation were efficient, it would not be possible to increase total medical benefits by taking some money away from one service, for example cancer chemotherapy, and spending it on another, say x-ray. Even superficial inspection of the situation in Britain indicates that this condition is not satisfied.

For lack of dialysis facilities, many people with chronic kidney failure die years earlier than necessary; yet relatively large expenditures prolong only briefly the lives of patients with metastatic cancer. Many hospitals lack CT scanners that could yield large medical benefits, whereas bone marrow transplantation for several hundred patients a year absorbs enough money to supply many of the missing CT scanners.

The disparities are explained in part by the inevitable irrationalities of any large bureaucracy. More important, they appear to reflect a series of social choices. Benefits that are not purely medical are being purchased.

In chapter 1 we listed some factors that we thought might influence the allocation of resources to health care in Britain. Here we explore them in the context of the various technologies we have studied. Obviously, our observations cannot be used to test the various hypotheses, but only to bolster or weaken their plausibility.* We do think that similar considerations would shape the pattern of health care in the

* If cost containment was not approached through revenue limits, but rather through some method of cost-sharing, we would expect these factors to play a different role, as discussed in the next chapter.

United States if rationing becomes prevalent here. Our readers will have to judge for themselves whether we have made a persuasive case that these hypotheses are likely to have general validity.

One class of conditions—acute, life-threatening illnesses—is largely exempt from the rationing process in Britain. Successful treatment of a brief but life-threatening illness yields a large payoff and thus encourages generous investment. Moreover, the way in which people with an acute illness usually enter the system facilitates their getting the most favorable treatment. Patients who arrive in an emergency room suffering from such acute conditions as diabetic coma, myocardial infarction, or trauma are promptly admitted to the hospital and given all available care. Once that step is taken, no effort is spared as long as there is even a remote chance of restoring normal or near normal health.

To test this perception, we asked several British physicians how they would handle an accident victim whose injuries we described. We based our query on a real case admitted to a large U.S. teaching hospital. Included in the case history was the estimate that the patient had one chance in a hundred of surviving and that the cost of his care could be expected to exceed $100,000. Confronted with one hundred similar cases, one would expect to save one life and to spend $10 million. Despite the limitations they face, the British physicians unanimously stated that they would have used all available resources just as their American counterparts had done. The same approach, we were told, is apparently not followed consistently with the elderly.

### Factors That Seem to Influence Allocations to Specific Technologies

It is apparent that the social influences on choices about levels of care often work in combination. A dread disease, cancer, is more likely to have organized advocates than one that causes less fear. On the other hand, no effective treatment is available for some cancers, and in many such cases survival is brief and the quality of life under therapy is low. In these cases, the power of cancer to attract resources will be offset by the near futility of treatment. In any specific instance, various forces will combine to determine the resources that will be committed to the particular technology. Disentangling these forces is a problem that defied any rigorous or formal analysis that we could devise. Failing that, however, we examined a variety of medical technologies to identify the principles that seem to govern the level of funding.

## Chronic Dialysis

As we have pointed out, the restriction of chronic dialysis in Britain causes many people to die earlier than they would if treatment were fully available to them. Many influences seem to contribute to this decision.

First, a commitment to treat all cases of chronic kidney failure would be extremely costly. If Britain dialyzed at the same rate as the United States, it would have to increase its total health expenditures by over 1 percent.[1] But this increment equals the real growth in all health expenditures planned for the next two years, according to Prime Minister Margaret Thatcher's budget request for 1983–84. Given this constraint, full-service dialysis could be provided only if large sacrifices were made in other areas of health care.

Second, hospital dialysis facilities can be limited in a fairly centralized way by controlling capital expenditure on equipment and by limiting numbers of qualified nurses and technicians. Thus doctors and patients alike perceive the limitation as an external constraint rather than as a personal choice.

Third, the general practitioner seldom has to face the constraint on dialysis. Given the rates at which kidney failure occurs, the typical family doctor may see only one case every two or three years.[2] Consultants see many more cases, of course, but their burden is lightened because general practitioners try not to refer patients who, their experience has taught them, are unlikely to be treated.

Finally, renal failure, which is usually manifested by weakness, nausea, and drowsiness, is neither a highly visible nor a dread disease. Furthermore, it is often accompanied by other diseases, such as long-standing diabetes, which can be used to rationalize the refusal of care.

## Hemophilia

Whatever can be said about chronic renal failure should be reversed for hemophilia, a disease that is treated as often and almost as intensively in Britain as in the United States. The illness is highly visible, and its symptoms alarm any observer. Treatment is conspicuously successful in the short run because patients feel almost entirely well between episodes. Capital investment required for treatment is minimal, and as we have mentioned, the total cost of treating all hemophiliacs, $30 million to $40 million a year, is one-tenth the potential cost of offering dialysis to all patients in chronic renal failure. Moreover, full treatment of hemophilia has the further benefit that it largely eliminates the potentially costly disabilities that result without it. Dialysis, on the other hand, may be perceived as a form of disability itself, because treatment immobilizes the patient several times a week and is accompanied by complications and discomforts of its own.

### Hip Replacement

Hip replacement is rationed in Britain, and the waiting lists are notoriously long, but in reality the British insert about 75 to 80 percent as many artificial hips per capita as Americans do. The total cost of this program is relatively high—about $100 million to $150 million a year.

Why is so much spent on hip replacement to reduce pain and improve mobility of the elderly, but so little on dialysis to save lives? First, hip replacement helps many people and at less total cost than dialysis. The typical dialysis patient is treated for several years or longer at an average cost of about $15,000 a year, whereas patients requiring hip replacement are treated once at a cost of only about $6,000. Moreover, those who undergo successful hip surgery enjoy a life of good quality, whereas dialysis is beset by complications and does not restore normal quality of life.

Finally, restoring mobility for the large number of patients with hip disease who otherwise would require extensive nursing care, either at home or in a public institution, avoids large indirect costs. By contrast, little would be saved by eliminating the modest expense of supporting the elderly, undialyzed renal failure patient during his brief terminal illness.

### Coronary Artery Surgery

The low rate of coronary artery surgery in Britain—10 percent of that in the United States—calls out for an explanation. Even if the American rate is too high, as seems likely, experts we have consulted believe that the British might do perhaps seven times as many cases a year with considerable medical profit.

Age hardly seems to be a factor. Hip surgery is provided to the same age group far more generously than is coronary artery surgery. Hip replacement, it is true, costs only one-half to two-thirds as much as a coronary bypass procedure, but this difference in cost does not seem to explain the large disparity in numbers of procedures performed. In 1977 some 27,000 hip replacements were performed on an estimated pool of 34,000 candidates, as contrasted with 3,000 bypass grafts for 20,000 highly suitable candidates for the surgery.

Two factors may account for this seeming anomaly. First, hip disease is more obvious than coronary artery disease. One can more easily apprehend the anguish of an elderly woman, bedridden or barely able to walk, than that of a middle-aged man who must walk slowly to avoid discomfort. Bypass surgery may also command fewer resources because the untreated patient with angina does not place the same burden on society's resources as do those with untreated hip disease. With medication alone, angina patients can usually look after their personal needs and remain mobile enough not to require nursing or other supportive care. Severe hip disease creates far greater demands.

## Radiotherapy

The quantity and quality of megavoltage radiotherapy in Britain and the United States are similar. Expenditures on radiotherapy in Britain are probably somewhat more than $100 million a year (based on an estimate of $500 million in the United States), a substantial sum in Britain's $13 billion hospital budget for 1980. Radiotherapy is the one expensive technology provided to the elderly for which demand is fully satisfied. Only hip replacement comes close.

Radiotherapy seems to enjoy a favored position for several reasons. One of them is historical. As one of the earliest of the expensive technologies, it came into use when resources were still relatively plentiful and thus was fully funded—an unlikely outcome today. Perhaps equally important, cancer is a dread disease. The special position of cancer in the public mind probably assures generous support for radiotherapy. This special concern is also seen in the large sums raised by such patient organizations as the Imperial Cancer Fund, which establishes professorships of oncology and supports other work on cancer.

## Cancer Chemotherapy

Cancer chemotherapy is administered to patients with potentially curable metastatic tumors at the same rate in Britain as in the United States. Here, age of the victims is an obvious reason; many of the potentially curable malignancies occur in relatively young people. A few thousand dollars may yield many years of life. Moreover, the total cost of the program is modest.

On the other hand, the British are much more conservative than Americans in their approach to tumors that respond poorly to chemotherapy, such as carcinomas of the pancreas or stomach. British oncologists say that in such cases the decision not to treat is made not on financial grounds but to spare their patients pointless suffering.

We could predict, however, that resource constraints would loom large if an expensive but effective form of chemotherapy could be developed for one or another of the common cancers. Tens of thousands of patients would be candidates, and the total cost would become large.

When asked what would happen under these circumstances, a leading British oncologist responded, "It is something I wake up screaming about. I suspect that not everybody who might benefit from [chemotherapy] would get it in practice. If you could cure every patient who has carcinoma of the colon, most of whom are going to be over sixty-five, over fifty-five anyway, I think we might find ourselves making value judgments about which to treat and which not to." As the case of chronic dialysis shows, even decisions to fund lifesaving care may become sensitive to the total cost of rendering such care.


### Bone Marrow Transplantation

Bone marrow transplantation is provided in Britain as frequently, per capita, as in the United States. Here the youth of the recipients and the often lifesaving nature of the treatment are important factors. Moreover, the diseases that are treated—chiefly leukemia and aplastic anemia—are visibly devastating. The aggregate cost is also relatively low because no more than a few hundred patients a year are suitable candidates for treatment. These influences work together to encourage full funding.


### CT Scanners

On its face, the relative lack of CT scanners in Britain is hard to explain. The technology is now recognized as a powerful, indeed revolutionary, diagnostic tool in many clinical situations. Nevertheless, the British spend only $20 million a year on CT scanning and have the capacity to perform only a fifth as many scans per capita as do

Americans. Most hospitals, including many major centers, do not have a machine, and their patients do not have ready access to a CT facility located elsewhere.

To reach a capacity comparable with that in the United States, Britain would have to spend only another $80 million. But the funds would have to come out of the limited resources available for capital expenditures on equipment and for the creation of staff positions. In other words, hospital physicians cannot simply commandeer a larger share of drugs, clinical space, or beds from the pool of general hospital space as with coronary bypass grafts or hip replacement. Obtaining new funds is also made more difficult by the absence of a constituency with a disease that depends on the machine. Most people do not know the circumstances under which a scan would benefit them and are unaware that they are being denied valuable care.

Nevertheless, the donation of scanners shows an increasing popular recognition of the shortage. Unless operating funds are also donated, the recipient hospital is forced to assume the ongoing costs of the machine, including its staffing.

### Total Parenteral Nutrition

The British spend only one-fourth as much per capita on TPN as the United States even though there are virtually no constraints on the physician's freedom to order this therapy. As with hemophilia, only pharmaceutical supplies and nursing care are needed. For this reason the therapist need not face the explicit constraints imposed on capital expenditures. Given these facts, one might expect that the use of total parenteral nutrition would grow rapidly throughout the British hospital system and that such use might quickly approach the level that we have observed in the United States. Why such convergence has not occurred is an interesting question.

The answer appears to be that British physicians as a group are skeptical of the value of TPN, which has been demonstrated to produce appreciable benefits only in a small minority of the people receiving it in the United States. Most British physicians have been circumspect about ordering the treatment and have acted to limit expenditures by colleagues who are viewed as TPN enthusiasts. This policy has not been undercut by the public because most people are almost unaware of TPN and unlikely to demand it.

Nevertheless, the British are spending a larger amount of money on TPN than on other procedures. We conclude that though clinical freedom to prescribe TPN is somewhat constrained by the British system of checks and balances, the system clearly does not prevent the medical entrepreneur from claiming substantial new resources under the umbrella of clinical freedom.

### Intensive Care Beds

With only one-tenth to one-fifth the number of intensive care beds available per capita as in the United States,[3] British physicians acknowledged that they could use more to medical advantage. But planners and physicians alike perceive the overall cost to be excessive. To reach parity with the United States, Britain would have to increase its total health care budget some 10 percent. One director of an intensive care unit in a teaching hospital said, "Such a move would be inappropriate given the enormous negative impact on other services that would have funds withdrawn from them. This [our unit] is about right and appropriate. It balances with the rest of what goes on around here. It would be crazy [to have more beds], you see, because it would be out of proportion to what we offer in the renal unit and what we offer anywhere else."

### Terminal Illness

We were told repeatedly that British physicians discontinue aggressive therapy for the terminally ill earlier than their American counterparts do. They also, and just as repeatedly, assert that they would elect to stop treatment earlier than Americans do, even if their resources were not constrained. We have no reason to dispute this claim, which undoubtedly reflects cultural traditions and ethical views.

On the other hand, the limitation on intensive care beds, the relative lack of facilities for chronic dialysis, and other constraints force British physicians to practice triage. They cannot routinely place a seventy-five-year-old patient with advanced metastatic cancer in an intensive care unit without an awareness that the bed is likely to be needed by a twenty-five-year-old accident victim. In the United States a physician who might explicitly agree with values expressed by his British colleague may nevertheless be allowed to avoid a hard decision by the sheer availability of the bed.

### Factors That Seem to Influence Resource Allocation

A set of general principles can be extracted from the representative technologies we have examined. Some reflect the influence of administrative arrangements on the allocation process. Others are an expression of society's value judgments or of attempts to make the most efficient use of resources.

### *Age*

If all other factors were held constant, we would expect less rationing of health care for children than for adults. Aggregate data support this prediction. Health expenditures per child in Britain are 119 percent of expenditures per prime age adult, whereas in the United States they are only 37 percent as much.[4]

These results are hardly surprising. Adults respond to sick children with strong emotions. Furthermore, care that saves a child's life or improves its quality yields benefits much longer than those same resources used on an older person.

The responsibilities of prime age adults as parents and earners sometimes override these considerations, but such offsetting factors seldom apply to the elderly. The low incidence of chronic dialysis among the elderly with renal failure dramatizes such discrimination. The limitation of resources allocated to the treatment of terminal illness is another expression of this bias.

### *Dread Disease*

Some diseases, depending on the culture and the historical moment, inspire more fear than others. Currently, the prime example is cancer. One might expect that such diseases would receive a disproportionate share of the available resources.

Such appears to be the case. Megavoltage radiotherapy is made available to all who can benefit from it, even if the expectation is palliation rather than cure. Moreover, cancer chemotherapy is provided to all in whom there is hope of prolonging life by as much as several years or an expectation of significant palliation of symptoms.

## Visibility of Illness

People do not like visible misery. They are made uncomfortable if they must watch severe and untreated suffering. The bleeding joints, swelling, and disabilities of hemophilia are likely to stir more feeling in bystanders than the silent pain of angina pectoris. It is thus not surprising that more support is allocated to clotting factors for hemophiliacs than to bypass surgery for angina patients, as is indeed the case in Britain.

## Advocacy

Organized advocates can try to use political pressure, publicity, or charity to obtain facilities and personnel for a particular service. Oddly enough, we found little evidence that advocacy plays an important role in shaping allocation decisions in Britain. Other than bone marrow transplantation, we have found no service significantly increased by the efforts of pressure groups. We suspect that in this regard the United States will prove to be quite different.

## Aggregate Cost

A service that is costly relative to the benefit it yields may still be provided if the total cost for all patients is fairly small. It may simply not be seen as worthwhile to enforce the general principles of rationing when the total cost of a program seems negligible. The full-scale treatment of hemophilia in Britain may be an example. Only about seventy-five new cases of hemophilia are diagnosed each year in Britain. At an annual cost of $10,000 to $20,000 each, this small number of patients appears to be exempted from rationing. It seems less likely that the same would be true if there were 25,000 new patients every year.

## Need for Capital Funds

The use of new technology can be controlled much more easily if it requires a large capital outlay than if it depends only on funds from the hospital's operating budget. A vivid contrast is provided by outlays on CT scanners as opposed to expenditures for total parenteral nutrition. Only about $10 million a year is committed to CT scanners, which have been installed in only a few hospitals, even though they could make an important contribution in any facility with more than 200 beds. By contrast, the benefit of total parenteral nutrition to most of the patients receiving it has not been well documented. But Britain spends as much on this service as on CT scanning. At least part of the reason, we surmise, is that total parenteral nutrition requires no appreciable capital outlay and can be allocated, case by case, at the discretion of individual physicians.

### Costs of Alternative Modes of Care

Our observations support the notion that a given therapy will be provided in larger quantity if the costs of not treating the patient exceed the costs of active intervention. This thesis gains compelling support from a comparison of coronary bypass surgery with hip replacement. The costs of each operation are similar, as are the ages of the patients, but hip replacements are done with far greater frequency. As we noted earlier, the much higher cost of caring for disabled patients with hip disease than for patients with angina seems likely to be the main determinant of the difference.

### Quality versus Quantity

Resources could be saved by reducing quality as well as quantity. Would it not therefore be sensible to dilute the quality of care in order to extend the quantity? In most instances the answer is no, and British decisions on resource allocation appear to reflect this judgment.

The British, as far as we could tell, and in the opinion of experts, maintain virtually the same standards of quality for CT scanning, coronary bypass surgery, hip replacement, cancer chemotherapy, and other such technologies as do Americans. In each of these instances, cutting corners would exact a heavy toll of bad outcomes and therefore make little sense. Instead, dollars are saved by reducing quantity.

In the few instances in which quality can be reduced without substantial harm, the British indeed have made the cuts. In diagnostic radiology, for example, the British use half as many films per examination as American radiologists. They also have older and much less sophisticated equipment and a less than optimal number of radiologists. The economies achieved in this way reduce the quality of information to some degree, but the dollars saved almost certainly can be applied to greater advantage elsewhere in the health care system.

Cost-saving is also achieved in radiotherapy by less than optimal staffing patterns. In radiotherapy, as in diagnostic radiology, such economies make sense because their effect on quality is viewed by experts as marginal.

A reduction in quality is also seen in hospital structure. Even though the United Kingdom has only slightly fewer beds per capita than the United States, it spends, on average, only $12 per capita annually on the construction of medical facilities while the United States spends $25.[5] Most hospitals in Britain were built before World War II and many before World War I. These older hospitals obviously do not offer the same amenities or the same efficiency in providing patient care as do new facilities. Given competing demands, however, the cost of replacing them would be excessive.

### Dealing with Resource Limits

Both doctors and patients in Britain have adjusted to severe resource limitations that are, as yet, unfamiliar to Americans. To maintain the social fabric while denying some patients useful and even lifesaving care is not easy. Patients and providers must live with the recognition that more money could be spent and that many patients would benefit, while nevertheless acknowledging that the opportunity costs, for British society as a whole, would be too large.

Supply limits on the health sector can come in many forms; the specific features will provoke specific behavioral responses. Nevertheless, most of the issues we consider here would, in our view, arise under any system that tried to limit expenditures.

### *The Physician's Way*

Resource limits set up a kind of competition for available resources. Doctors increase control over resources by taking them away from other doctors and their patients, but the extent to which this game can be played is limited. For this reason the British physician often appears to rationalize, or at least to redefine, medical standards so that he can deal more comfortably with resource constraints.

RATIONALIZATION. Resource limits put doctors in a position that many of them find awkward. Trained to treat illness, they find they are unable to provide all the care from which their patients might derive some positive medical benefit. Even if such limits accurately reflect the social or political judgment that the expected benefit of care is worth less than the cost, balancing of costs and benefits is not part of the training or professional ethics of most physicians. Wherever possible, therefore, British doctors seem to seek medical justification for decisions forced on them by resource limits. Doctors gradually redefine standards of care so that they can escape the constant recognition that financial limits compel them to do less than their best.

By various means, physicians and other health care providers try to make the denial of care seem routine or optimal. Confronted by a person older than the prevailing unofficial age cutoff for dialysis, the British GP tells the victim of chronic renal failure or his family that nothing can be done except to make the patient as comfortable as possible in the time remaining. The British nephrologist tells the family of a patient who is difficult to handle that dialysis would be painful and burdensome and that the patient would be more comfortable without it; or he tells the resident alien from a poor country that he should return home, to be among family and friends who speak the same language—where, as it happens, the patient will die because dialysis is unavailable. Cardiologists focus on the relatively narrow class of cases in which coronary artery surgery demonstrably increases survival rates, or in which anginal pain is disabling, and downplay the cases in which pain is less severe.

In each instance physicians are asserting that the treatment is *medically* optimal or very close to optimal, that patients denied care or provided alternative forms of care because of budget limits lose essentially nothing of medical significance. For the undialyzed patient with renal failure who dies, for the victim of angina who must bear pain, or for the patient with head injuries whose diagnosis is wrong because a CT scanner was unavailable, this view is unpersuasive even if the underlying judgment that resources must be limited is correct. But it enables doctors to avoid the painful realization that they are doing less than the best for the patient.

Thus it is clear that not all British doctors believe they are providing all potentially beneficial care to their patients. Many realize, according to one consultant, that they are acting as society's agent in rationing care. Others may sometimes believe the medical rationalizations for budget limits and sometimes see through them. Another consultant spoke to us about the process: "The sense that I have is that there are many situations where resources are sufficiently short so that there must be decisions made as to who is treated. Given that circumstance, the physician, in order to live with himself and to sleep well at night, has to look at the arguments for not treating a patient. And there are always some—social, medical, whatever. In many instances he heightens, sharpens, or brings into focus the negative component in order to make himself and the patient comfortable about not going forward. He states the reason for not going forward in medical terms. . . but that formulation in many instances is in no small part conditioned by the fact that there really aren't enough resources to treat everybody, and there is a kind of rationalization which is, perhaps, influenced by resource constraints."

Although most British doctors would like to deploy more resources than are now available, they seem to recognize that their country is not rich enough to provide all the care that might be beneficial. In responding to a question about whether he thought more beds in his hospital should be devoted to intensive care, a doctor in charge of an intensive care unit at one of London's leading teaching hospitals summed up in this way: "No, everybody would get bored stiff and the place would be half-empty. It would be a great big sham. It is empire building to blow it up that big. You would set your threshold here much lower. It has to be appropriate to the surroundings. Now what we have by your standards is way short of the mark. It would be too small in America, but if you took this unit and put it down in the middle of Sri Lanka or India, it would stick out like a sore thumb. It would be an obscene waste of money."

Once such a concession to economic reality is made, doctors prefer to find medical rationales for what is fiscally necessary. They can then at least halfway believe they are giving their patients the best care, all things considered, that it is possible for them to give.

ATTEMPTS TO EXPLOIT CLINICAL FREEDOM. The British profess that each doctor, in consultation with his patient, should be free to determine the best method of diagnosis and treatment and that this decision is not to be subjected to second guessing, except in egregious circumstances and then only by medical colleagues or the courts. This principle derives from the importance of factors specific to each case in prescribing treatment and reflects the need for doctors to make dozens of choices a day quickly and decisively.

Under the rubric of clinical freedom a physician can sometimes take advantage of the system by diverting resources to patients in whom he is interested. The prodigality of one physician in treating his patients obviously reduces the resources available to other doctors. When such a situation is recognized, other doctors intervene.

The British system is almost ideally constructed to handle the threats to budget limits from exploitation of the commitment to clinical freedom. Most of the power over each hospital's budget rests in the hands of the hospital's consultants. This small staff of senior doctors is employed on salary under lifetime tenure. Although the outcome of debates about the allocation of the hospital's budget affects the resources available to each consultant, the debates are not shadowed by personal financial consequences for any of them. Negotiations are said to be marked by compromise and trade-offs born of the recognition that each participant must spend all or most of his professional life in the company of the same colleagues.

For the most part these debates concern questions of capacity and maintenance—what equipment to buy, what rehabilitations to seek, what staff to hire, what vacancies to leave unfilled—and do not normally involve the medical practice of individual physicians. Only rarely does an innovative and expensive practice undertaken by a particular physician pose a threat to a hospital's budget.

The introduction of new chemotherapeutic agents to treat cancer created such a problem for one leading British cancer hospital. The introduction and aggressive use of total parenteral nutrition caused budgetary difficulties in still another hospital. In one health district where financial resources were meager, an increase in the implantation of cardiac pacemakers generated unanticipated costs large enough to throw a balanced budget into deficit. In each such case the doctors responsible for the high expenditures were apprised of the problem, and through informal talks expansion of the new activities was curbed. In the case of the cancer drug, new funds were found to cover the jump in expenditures, but the hospital was instructed to avoid such overruns in the future. Negotiations effectively capped the budget for TPN. Thus threats to the hospital's budget were negotiated away.

The clinical freedom of the general practitioner working outside the hospital is not a serious threat to the budget. Although his right to prescribe is theoretically unlimited, he has little effective call on resources, because he does not prescribe costly drugs or have direct access to expensive diagnostic techniques. Health authorities have periodically reviewed the wisdom of continuing the GP's unlimited power to prescribe, but have concluded that imposing the limits was not desirable.[6]

SHORT-CIRCUITING DELAYS. A major consequence of limited resources in British hospital care is that familiar British phenomenon, the queue. Except in emergencies, care may be delayed for considerable periods of time. The concerned physician can exploit several mechanisms to shorten the wait. The general practitioner who feels that a patient should be seen by a consultant without a long delay knows that he is more likely to get his patient seen by telephoning the consultant than by writing a letter. If he wants even faster action, the GP can stipulate that his patient is too sick to travel and must be seen at home. Domiciliary visits, or house calls, result in extra income and are reportedly made promptly. GPs on occasion reportedly exaggerate a patient's immobility to get him seen sooner. The number of domiciliary visits increased about one-third during the 1970s.[7] Although these methods of cutting delays are sometimes useful, they do not, in the view of British clinicians, play an important role in breaking through the constraints of the system.

THE PROBLEM OF SAYING NO. British physicians often have to refuse certain patients treatment; the older patient who is a candidate for chronic dialysis is the prime example. Saying no to such a patient will always be difficult. But the local internist who convinces himself that the patient is unsuitable because he is "a bit crumbly" can say no with less discomfort.

For many older patients with renal failure, the local physician does not even raise the possibility of dialysis. In other circumstances, however, he says that dialysis does not seem to be indicated. Because of the respect that most patients have for physicians, the doctor's recommendations are usually followed with little complaint.

The local physician's role as gatekeeper explains a puzzling phenomenon observed at several dialysis centers. Early on we asked directors of several centers how they turned away the many older patients referred to them for treatment. To our surprise they said they rarely had such a problem. Only later did it become clear that older patients are seldom referred to dialysis centers because the referring physician is well aware that they could not be accommodated. By not referring the patient, the doctor spares the nephrologist from having to say no and the patient and family a painful rejection. He also avoids the need to face the rejected patient and relatives.

## Safety Valves for the Patient

No general budget ceiling on medical care, even one set by the most democratic of procedures, can match the diverse preferences of all people subject to it. Officials interested in setting limits on medical expenditures must therefore decide not only how much to allocate to health but also what to do about efforts by private citizens to spend their own funds on medical care. The two principal channels for such expenditures in Britain are charitable gifts and private medical care. In computing taxable income, British taxpayers may deduct gifts to hospitals or other public health facilities, but the tax law does not permit the deduction of private health expenditures or health insurance premiums.

The ability of British citizens to make gifts to health facilities and to buy health care outside the National Health Service is a safety valve that allows people to indulge preferences for more or different health care than that provided by the NHS. It also means that excessively stringent limits on NHS expenditures threaten the survival of the health service as a vehicle for elective health care; if limits become too tight, people can "go private."

The deductibility of gifts to private charitable organizations and the regulatory policies that permit NHS doctors to spend two-elevenths of their time practicing privately have an important indirect bearing on popular attitudes toward the budget limits imposed on the National Health Service. The more attractive the choices are outside the NHS, the less burdensome will be the budget limits constraining it.[8]

CHARITY. Charity plays a minor part in British medicine as a whole but is significant in selected fields. A few large hospitals retain endowments from pre-NHS days. Certain kinds of medical equipment, notably CT scanners, have been purchased largely out of donated funds. Private funds have endowed senior consultancies in certain fields, notably oncology, to increase the prestige and visibility of such specialties. District health officials differ in the degree to which they seek charitable contributions to supplement NHS funds, but some report that such gifts have been important, particularly during the recent period of slow growth in NHS spending.

Some lessons emerge from these gifts. First, donors are reported to give equipment or a facility more willingly than to pay for its continued operation and maintenance. For this reason gifts have often enticed or pressured authorities into changing their priorities. The gift of a CT scanner, unaccompanied by funds for staff, supplies, and maintenance, thus burdens the budget of the district, area, or region where the scanner is located. Endowing a chair for a professor may entail the complementary hiring of junior doctors and other support staff and necessitate assignment to the professor of a reasonable number of beds to which he will have admitting privileges. These expenses usually fall on the NHS budget. For these reasons, both health authorities and the universities have begun to decline offers that do not include funds for operating or ancillary expenses. Second, insofar as health authorities anticipate gifts, they can divert their own resources to other purposes. In that way gifts do not change priorities but rather augment total health spending. Faced with limited resources, budget planners can shortchange activities for which charitable gifts can be anticipated or elicited. Though we have no evidence, we suspect that the NHS would have bought more CT scanners than it did if private donations had not partially filled the gap and if further donations were not anticipated.

THE PRIVATE SECTOR. When the public sector does not provide all the health care demanded at zero price, patients must decide whether to seek through other channels care that they are denied within the controlled system. Their willingness to do so depends on two considerations: how highly they value the curtailed services and how much they must personally pay for them.

Patients are well situated to gain access to care if they are informed and aggressive and if they have the financial means, through direct payment or insurance, to buy care or amenities in short supply within the controlled system. For example, patients willing to see consultants as private patients are more likely to receive care inside the NHS for diseases with long waiting lists, such as hip replacement and hernias.

Until the late 1970s, however, private health care remained a tiny, though growing, part of British health care. As indicated in chapter 2, the private sector is now growing rapidly and provides a significant part of some forms of health care. Thus a patient facing a long wait for elective surgery in an aging NHS hospital may instead choose prompt treatment in a new private hospital where he can have such amenities as a private room. Moreover, the NHS provides backup protection against serious complications; patients who prove to need specialized care unavailable in a private hospital can be moved to an NHS facility. For example, if a major cardiac or pulmonary problem or serious infection develops after hip surgery, the patient will be transferred immediately.

But the private sector is unlikely to provide the high-priced and sophisticated care that is currently supplied almost exclusively by the NHS. First, such care depends on highly specialized equipment and laboratories and on junior physicians to provide twenty-four-hour care, all of which involve high overhead expenses. Such costly care can therefore be sustained only if the demand is high. Unless shortages become pervasive enough to drive a critical mass of British patients into the private sector for such services, private medicine will be unable to afford to offer the full range of service required for high-quality tertiary care.

Second, insurance coverage for such care is unlikely to develop in any large way. People at low risk of needing elaborate and costly care are unlikely to pay premiums for private insurance to cover the costs of procedures, such as dialysis, that might have to be obtained outside the system. But if only high-risk people sign up, the insurance cannot be profitably underwritten. Thus, as a case in point, virtually no dialysis in Britain is performed outside the National Health Service.

WORKING THE SYSTEM. Though most British patients are said to take the word of their physicians on a course of action (or nonaction), some do not passively accept a denial of care. Such people have several strategies open to them if they wish to press forward within the system. A patient can ask his physician to arrange for a second opinion. In most instances, we are told, this kind of referral is provided without protest. Or the patient may try to gain access to specialized services for which he or she might have previously been deemed "unsuitable" by going to a hospital emergency room, even that of a major university hospital. The emergency room also provides access to primary care services that are scarce outside office hours.

Alternatively, on rare occasions the patient may penetrate the referral barrier by going directly to the clinic of a specialist. One leading nephrologist told us, for example, that a patient who sits down in the waiting room will probably be seen and a slot found for him in the dialysis program. A cancer expert at one of the main British centers emphasized how difficult it is to refuse care to a patient who appears at the doorstep. The key to turning down the patient "is not to get eyeball to eyeball with him because if you do there is no way you can actually say no."

Aggressive behavior by a patient seeking care is now manageable. Patients normally fear alienating their GP by trying to circumvent his decisions. But consultants express some fear that the regular system in which the GP or local consultant determines who will be seen in referral could break down if too many patients go to hospital emergency rooms and clinics from which they cannot be turned away. Clearly the GP and the local consultant can act as gatekeepers only because few patients go outside of channels.

EXPLOITING GEOGRAPHY. Shortages are worse in some places than in others. For example, waiting times for hip replacement vary widely across regions.[9] Administrative impediments do not hinder patients who wish to travel to an uncrowded hospital for care, but most patients are reluctant to leave familiar surroundings and the emotional support provided by friends and relatives. As a result, few patients travel to find short queues.

### Why Malpractice Litigation Does Not Mobilize Resources

In principle, malpractice suits could be used to put pressure on the government to expand medical services. For example, patients with head injuries who are mishandled for lack of CT scanners might sue both physicians and the local hospital authorities. If costly awards against the government were to result, the government might find it cheaper to provide more CT scanners than to continue paying damages.

In practice, however, there are few malpractice suits. The cost of litigation is high. The plaintiff must pay his lawyer on an hourly basis rather than arrange a contingency fee. Should he lose, the plaintiff must also pay the defendant's costs—typically, even as of 1971, $7,500 to $25,000. The legal aid scheme entitles plaintiffs to government aid if annual disposable income is below $8,800 and capital is below $5,500. But administrative obstacles to obtaining aid and required out-of-pocket payments, which can reach nearly $4,000, deter litigation.[10]

Thus, not surprisingly, in 1982 the annual premium charged by the Medical Defence Union, the largest and oldest of Britain's three malpractice insurers, was only about $250—a reflection of the low frequency of claims and awards. In the twenty-five years from 1947 to 1972, only 2,809 malpractice claims were brought.[11]

Another sort of suit is possible, under the National Health Services Act of 1977, which stipulates that "the Secretary of State is under a duty to provide services to such an extent that he considers necessary to meet all reasonable requirements."[12] Patients or doctors might bring an action to make the Secretary do his duty under the law, that is to require the central government to provide appropriate facilities, as they see it. So far, no such action has been initiated.

## Political and Social Responses to Resource Constraints

We have found only two recent examples of complaints in the press that adequate medical care is not being provided to the British people. One concerns the shortage of dialysis facilities, and the other a presumed shortage of facilities for bone marrow transplantation.

In the case of dialysis, the press generated enough pressure on the government to cause the minister of health to respond in a letter to the London *Sunday Mirror* (March 30, 1981). The minister acknowledged that many deaths had occurred because facilities were not available and pinpointed money as the issue. His suggestion that private charity close the gap was greeted derisively by the media. Earlier the London *Times* (March 20, 1980) had printed an article called "1000 Kidney Patients Die Because Treatment Unavailable," in which a leading nephrologist was quoted as saying: "Some of us have to tell lies to older patients, partly to make the patients more comfortable and partly to make ourselves more comfortable. We have to say to them that their hearts are too dodgy to stand the strain of dialysis. But we are getting fed up with telling lies."

Although this view is shared by many nephrologists, we were told that many senior physicians in other specialties consider kidney transplantation and dialysis medical frills, maintaining that the funds could be used to greater advantage for other kinds of treatment. Thus any pressure from the media will probably not lead to much increase in resources available for dialysis at the local level, where the process of allocation usually occurs. Only if the national government directly allocated funds for dialysis would much more money be forthcoming. The British Renal Association, a patient-dominated organization, is fostering such a policy, but so far to little effect.

Bone marrow transplantation has also become politically sensitive and controversial even though the National Health Service seems to have fully met the demand for the treatment of people with matched sibling donors.[13] On the other hand, an article in the *Lancet* reported in 1981: "Lack of funding for bone marrow transplants, leading apparently to the deaths of many children who could have been saved if more cash were available for transplant programmes, has had much publicity lately."[14] This lament apparently derives from an article in the *Times Health Supplement* (November 12, 1981), which reported that ninety-seven children had died while waiting for bone marrow transplants. The *Times* reported later that within twenty-four hours of publication of the article the prime minister announced a special inquiry.

How do experts in bone marrow transplantation feel about the public claim that not enough is being done and that many lives are being lost? One such physician described the article in the *Lancet* as "a piece of political writing not deserving serious consideration." The long-term effect of media involvement on funding for BMT remains uncertain.

### Summary

The patterns of behavior described in this chapter are the natural responses of patients and providers to a system of medical care characterized by excess demand. All the British responses, of course, depend to some degree on British history, politics, social relations, and national psychology. Even so, we believe that the general nature of the British responses to budget limits would be apparent within the United States as well.

British experience suggests the following generalizations about the kinds of medical care likely to be curtailed most by budget limits.

—Services that depend on dedicated capital equipment and highly specialized staff will be cut far more than services that can be provided by regular hospital personnel and ordinary drugs and supplies. Decisions on the former confront physicians with a fait acccompli to which they must adjust; decisions on the latter require doctors to deny care to specific patients.

—Arcane services for which the need is not clearly evident to patients, such as total parenteral nutrition or CT scans, will be curtailed more readily than services for which the need is clear and inescapable.

—Services for the elderly are more likely to be curtailed than services for children or young adults, though even services for children will be curtailed if the cost of treatment per patient is very high.

—The treatment of cancer is a special case, probably because of its special character as a dread disease. Chemotherapy will probably be provided for all cases of metastatic disease where there is a potential for cure. Similarly megavoltage radiation therapy will be provided for both curative and palliative therapy to all patients regardless of age. Bone marrow transplantation will also probably be carried out at a high rate, in part because of the fear cancer engenders, in part because patients tend to be children and young adults and the payoff to successful treatment high.

—More generally, constraints will probably cause greater curtailment, other things equal, of methods of treatment or diagnosis that claim a large share of the health budget than of those that claim a small share. Thus when and if a successful artificial heart is developed, at a cost now put at $100,000 a patient, the fact that heart disease is the most frequent cause of death will force a budget-constrained system to ration its use quite ruthlessly. Heart and liver transplantation may also be sharply limited.

—The higher the quality of life after successful treatment, the smaller will be the reduction of care under budget limits.

The British physician and patient have developed many methods for dealing with resource constraints, all of which make life under budget constraints more tolerable. The British physician often seems to adjust his indications for treatment to bring into balance the demand for care and the resources available to provide it. This kind of rationalization preserves as much as possible the feeling that all care of value is being provided. Most of the British doctors whom we pressed, however, admit that though they would like to have more resources than are now available, they understand that competing demands make it impossible to do everything of medical benefit.

Some physicians try to exploit, on their patient's behalf, the right of the physician to order from the pharmacy without restriction. Large expenditures on total parenteral nutrition and on certain drugs for the treatment of cancer have sometimes resulted, but a system of checks and balances within the hospital has curtailed expenditures viewed as excessive.

Most patients in Britain appear willing to accept their doctor's word if he says that no further treatment of a particular disease is warranted. This passivity may stem from lack of knowledge about possible treatments or simply from a patient's respect for the physician's authority.

Safety valves exist that allow the persistent patient to circumvent the limitations imposed by the National Health Service. Patients can pay to see a consultant and also to get a pay bed in a NHS hospital, thereby jumping the usual queues for elective surgery. Elective care is also available without delay, and with many amenities, at private hospitals. The growth of private insurance in recent years shows that such care is increasingly valued. But serious, acute illnesses are still cared for almost exclusively in NHS hospitals.

Patients who refuse to take no for an answer when specialized care is denied them can often "work the system" successfully. By presenting themselves directly to a specialized unit, they make it difficult for the physician in charge to turn them away. Patients also have the option of going to a region other than their own where waiting lists are shorter, though few seem to take advantage of that option.

The British legal system does not provide a useful mechanism for pressing the government to allocate more resources to the health care system. It is difficult to bring pressure on the government through malpractice claims because of the financial impediments to suit.

In sum, our explanation for the behavior of the British health care system in allocating resources is consistent with both intuition and common sense. We also believe that the way patients and physicians have adapted to the system in Britain has important implications for the United States. The serious legal, medical, and ethical problems that will arise in the United States when patients or their families refuse to accept the medical consequences of budget constraints are a subject for the next chapter.

_chapter eight_ **Rationing Hospital Care in the United States**


       The cost of health care in the United States will continue growing for the foreseeable future. The technological revolution that helped boost real per capita medical expenditures 5 percent a year from 1965 to 1980 shows no sign of abating. During the next two decades the population aged seventy-five and older will rise 70 percent. And health care is what economists call a superior good, one that claims an increasing part of the consumer's dollar as his or her income rises. Economic growth, therefore, will tend to boost the share of national income devoted to health care. According to actuarial projections, the cost of hospital insurance under medicare, 2.97 percent of the social security wage base in 1982, will more than double by 2005, to 6.29 percent, and nearly quadruple by 2035, to over 11 percent.[1]

       If Americans could be confident that the expected incremental benefit of all medical care they buy exceeds the incremental cost of those services, the growth in medical expenditures, like similar past increases in spending on automobiles, television, and computers, would be a measure of the superior capacity of new commodities to satisfy consumer wants. But the system of third-party reimbursement precludes such rosy interpretations. Because care is essentially free when demanded, incentives encourage the provision of all care that produces positive benefits whatever the cost. Combined with scientific ingenuity, this system has led not only to dramatic advances in diagnosis and therapy but also to the use of technologically sophisticated and costly methods to provide medical care that is sometimes of slight value. Small increases in the certainty of diagnoses often come at great cost. Moreover, the ability to extend life during terminal illnesses and the difficulty of stopping treatment once it is begun create incentives for the provision of care that often reduces the quality of the dying patient's remaining life.

The problem that all developed nations face is how to alter the behavior of providers and patients so that expenditures are curtailed on care that, in some sense, is worth less than it costs. The British have addressed this question directly. For several reasons they have been able to hold expenditures on medical care well below those in the United States and other industrial nations. As discussed in the previous chapter, we judge that it would be possible for the British to achieve somewhat better medical results by reallocating resources. However, we believe that the actual patterns of expenditure are quite reasonable if one takes social considerations into account.

U.S. policy toward the growth of medical expenditures has been piecemeal and irregular. Legislation has required purchasers of costly equipment and other facilities to demonstrate unmet demand or otherwise to justify proposed expenditures. The Nixon administration briefly imposed direct price controls on hospitals. Successive administrations have proposed longer-term limits. Several states and smaller entities have put limits of various kinds on the growth of hospital revenues. But these steps have had little overall effect on health expenditures.

The question of how large health expenditures should be will not go away. Rather, technologic change, an aging population, and the rising demand for health care flowing from higher incomes will make the question even more pressing.

### Constraints and Their Consequences

We think it highly probable that states and the federal government will increase their efforts to hold down hospital expenditures and other medical outlays. Proposals for federal legislation and state actions suggest that policymakers will largely rely on prospective reimbursement to encourage hospital administrators and physicians to seek less costly ways to provide health care.

In 1983 Congress established a dramatically new plan that uses prospective reimbursement for all medicare payments. Under this program the payment to a hospital would be predetermined for each of many diagnostic related groupings (DRGs). The hospital would be at risk for any expenditure greater than that authorized for the particular illness.

The most sweeping initiative by a state occurred in 1982 in Massachusetts, where hospitals were mandated to slow the growth of spending by adhering to a strict, predetermined formula. Over a five-year period a successful program of this sort could well reduce expenditures by some 35 or 40 percent below what otherwise would be expected. And also in 1982 California implemented a program to control medicaid costs that requires hospitals to bid for a contract under which the hospital provides all services to medicaid patients at a flat daily rate.[2]

These signs suggest that limits on reimbursement will be the principal instrument for controlling expenditures. We cannot forecast to what extent other instruments will be used—regulations to curtail purchases of buildings and equipment, reductions in benefits under public programs, and changes in tax laws or other measures to make patients more sensitive to the price of health care—but we do not believe they will be the dominant instruments.

Obviously the problems that will arise under budget limits and the responses of different groups to them will depend on how severe the limits are and on the political and economic situation at the time they are imposed. We have no way of knowing whether ceilings would be low and hard to avoid or high and easy to avoid. Past experience with regulation in the United States suggests the likelihood of "regulatory capture"—the infiltration of the regulatory mechanism by people sympathetic to the regulated industry—and attendant relaxation of regulatory controls.[3] Were this to happen to the organizations responsible for establishing budget limits, high and permeable ceilings might result. For these reasons, one cannot predict in detail how various groups will respond to budget limits or even whether the limits will be practicable.

Nevertheless, some results can be foreseen with reasonable confidence. Providers are likely to seek ways of escaping the constraints, and patients of obtaining the care they might otherwise be denied. If financial limits prevent the provision of some beneficial care, certain patients and illnesses will probably fare better than others. Demand will be fully met in some cases; in others, constraints on expenditures will reduce either quality or quantity.

## Means of Enforcement

A variety of instruments is available to governments in the United States to enforce both overall budget limits, like those in Britain, and such partial limits as diagnostic related groupings.

The federal government could deny reimbursement under medicare or medicaid to hospitals that violated federal or state regulations, the enforcement mechanism proposed by both the Ford and Carter administrations. It could use the Internal Revenue Code to enforce or promote limits. At present, employers may deduct the cost of health insurance premiums paid on behalf of employees, and the employees are not required to pay tax on the value of such insurance. The law could be amended to deny employers the deduction or to require employees to treat the premiums as taxable income if the insurance payments violate a budget limit. Authorization to buy expensive medical equipment might be granted only to hospitals that complied with budget limits. States could enforce budget limits by using their authority to regulate hospitals and insurance companies. Alone or together with the federal government they could effectively prevent the existence of health facilities not subject to revenue constraints. Indeed, a central regulatory and political question will be whether such providers should be allowed to exist.

Steps could also be taken to limit reimbursement of doctors. The fact that most doctors are paid on a fee-for-service or piece-rate basis, rather than by salary, complicates this task. Means of control exist, but they may be hard to enforce. Physicians' fees could be included, for example, under a payment system based on diagnostic related groupings. Just as the hospital is paid a fixed amount for removing a gall bladder or treating the victim of a heart attack, the doctor could be limited to a fixed fee for each service.

### Possible Savings without Denying Benefits

Limitations on hospital expenditures will end some activities that yield no medical benefit but consume resources. If budget limits caused the elimination only of such services, they would be painless. Despite naive hopes, however, medical spending can be reduced little by eliminating such pure waste.

Among the targets overoptimistically identified as important sources of potential saving are duplicated hospital facilities. But a study of the four kinds of facilities most often singled out as costly and redundant—CT scanners, open-heart surgery and cardiac catheterization units, megavoltage radiation units, and general hospital beds—indicated that in 1975 no more than $1 billion, about 2 percent of hospital costs, would have been saved if every unit met standards put forward by the Department of Health and Human Services.[4] These savings would not reduce subsequent growth of outlays.

Savings from eliminating duplication would be small because most facilities already operate at or above guideline minimums. Furthermore, care provided to patients transferred to a consolidated hospital is often almost as costly as care provided in an underused hospital. Savings from a reduction of duplication in such facilities as laboratories and laundries are unlikely to be significant. A reduced number of facilities also forces some patients to travel farther and wait longer to get care. And because hospitals would fight closures, substantial regulatory costs would be incurred as hospitals turned to regulation agencies and the courts. As a result, the net saving would be much smaller than the $1 billion that would be theoretically achievable.[5]

A shift of care from the inpatient to the outpatient sector seems equally unpromising. A critical review of the literature provides little or no evidence that appreciable savings have been achieved. Moreover, a careful theoretical analysis indicates that substituting outpatient for inpatient services would not substantially reduce total hospital expenditures.[6]

Cutting back on inefficient use of people and equipment will also not save much. Administrative inefficiencies will undoubtedly decrease as providers become cost conscious. Numbers of laboratory tests and x-rays that have no value will be reduced, but even a 25 percent reduction would save relatively little, because marginal costs are low. Preadmission screening and shorter stays can also cut costs. Cutting these inefficiencies would probably not have a major effect on hospital costs, because increases in such inefficiencies from year to year are not responsible for the rapid growth in hospital spending.

### The Need to Give Up Benefits

Four factors explain rising hospital expenditures: rising incomes, the growth of third-party coverage, technological advances, and the aging of the population. The spread of third-party coverage through private insurance and public programs has freed more patients and physicians from the need to worry about cost at the time of care. Growth of the population, in general, and of the elderly, in particular, has contributed to an increase of 2 percent a year in hospital admissions.[7] The most important factor, however, has been technological change, which has increased the number of beneficial services. Hip replacements, chronic dialysis, coronary bypass surgery, and CT scanners are but a few of the advances of the past decade. Waiting in the technologic wings are other

expensive procedures: the highly publicized artifical heart, liver transplantation, costly successors to CT scanners, artificial skin for the
treatment of burns, methods of genetic engineering, and treatment for
cancer with antibodies specific to the patient's malignant cells. Any
appreciable restraint on expenditures will be accomplished only at the
price of denying medical benefits. A large proportion of any forgone
care is likely to be on that part of the benefit curve where benefits are
low relative to costs.[8]

The new technology of the last decade provides a wealth of evidence
supporting this prediction. Take, for instance, the use of the CT scanner
for a patient who has unexplained dizziness or headaches that the doctor
feels are almost certainly caused by tension. Because the likelihood of
finding a treatable lesion by means of a scan is low, the cost of the many
studies required to find the one patient with a lesion is high. Moreover,
as new noninvasive methodologies, such as CT scanners, have replaced
risky or painful techniques, the pool of patients who are candidates for
study has expanded. Doctors are no longer forced to weigh the risk and
discomfort of invasive procedures against the potential gain of information; consequently, any return greater than zero becomes medically
justified.[9]

Expensive treatments, such as intensive care, have added to the high-
cost, low-benefit problem. In many cases admission to the intensive care
unit only marginally reduces risk but adds greatly to expenditure. Dialysis
can also be a relatively high-cost, low-benefit investment; for example,
when treatment of chronic renal failure is undertaken to extend briefly
the life of a blind diabetic with gangrene of the legs who has already had
several heart attacks.

Advocates of health maintenance organizations hold that HMOs hold
the answer to spiraling medical costs. They point out that HMOs deliver
health care for 18 to 47 percent less than fee-for-service providers are
able to do.[10] Outpatient services are equally costly, but hospitalization
rates of HMOs are far lower than those of fee-for-service providers. The
reasons for the difference remain in dispute. The age of patients, their
attitudes, the style of practice of participating physicians all may play a
role, but they do not explain all the difference. At least part of the savings
seems to come from the fact that HMOs admit fewer "discretionary" or
"unnecessary" cases than fee-for-service providers do. Advocates of
HMOs argue that these savings entail little or no loss of medical benefit.
It is also possible that HMOs undertreat some cases because of the
financial incentives to do so.

Even if HMOs offer real savings, however, they are not the long-run answer to the problem addressed in this book, the tendency of medical expenditures generating benefits worth less than costs to grow rapidly. First, only a minority of patients elect to join HMOs. Although tax provisions reduce the incentives of patients to seek the savings that health maintenance organizations make possible,[11] there is no evidence that many patients would abandon fee-for-service care even if the tax laws were changed.

Second, and more subtle, health maintenance organizations are subject to the same technological forces as other providers are. Even though it would be a notable achievement if savings like those claimed for HMOs could be achieved throughout the medical care system, the steady increase in expenditures on new technologies will persist. Some of those expenditures will be fully justified, but some will be of little or no value. If it were possible to reduce "unnecessary admissions" in the fee-for-service sector enough to bring its expenditures down to those of HMOs, the growth of outlays might be reduced for several years. But if underlying technology continued to drive up outlays at the same rate as in the past, the respite would be temporary. To summarize: even if HMOs continue to grow, long-term cost containment will require that hard choices be made about who gets what kind of care.

## Problems in Implementing Limits

The nature of the response of the American hospital system to limits on reimbursement tight enough to reduce quality or quantity of care would depend on the character of the limits. Using diagnostic related groupings as a way to control the cost per admission clearly illustrates this point.

DRGs provide the payment of a fixed amount per admission according to the categories into which a patient falls. Payment is based on several cost indicators, including the primary diagnosis, the secondary diagnosis, the age of the patient, and such aspects of care as surgical procedures. Game playing can pervert this process, however. The system encourages surgery and other procedures that lead to higher payments. Further, DRGs encourage hospitals to manipulate the sequence of diagnoses or otherwise classify an illness in the most financially advantageous way. Limitations on expenditures per admission, such as those imposed by DRGs, encourage admissions of easy cases previously handled on an outpatient basis. They also encourage hospitals to shorten lengths of stay and to release and readmit patients for further therapy. Limitations on payments per patient day, rather than per admission, would also encourage admissions of easy cases but would induce hospitals to lengthen rather than shorten stays, because the last days of care are usually the cheapest.

British-style limitations on annual expenditures would raise different problems because such controls require complex formulas to adjust for wage rates, population growth, age structure, and so on. Hospitals assigned a given revenue ceiling would complain that they were being treated inequitably or that due process had not been followed and would bring their complaints before the appropriate regulatory agency. They would plead special circumstances—replacement of an old boiler, an epidemic, a special wage settlement—to gain extra allowance through appeal or negotiations. Indeed, prospective reimbursement in New York State has led to just such a flood of appeals and court cases.[12] Whether the program was administered by states or the national government would affect the problems that arose in metropolitan areas covering two or more states.

Reaction of hospital staff would also help to determine whether these controls will be politically sustainable and technically efficient. Whether controls are introduced with the cooperation or over the resistance of physicians, unions of hospital workers, and other such groups would determine whether those groups became agents for enforcing limits or centers of resistance to them.

### Patients, Providers, and Budget Limits

Overall budget limits of the kind enforced in Britain would change almost everyone's relation to the health system. The affected groups include patients in general and the elderly in particular, physicians and other health care providers, organized labor, business, and lawyers. And suppliers of all the commodities that hospitals use, such as drugs and equipment, would find sales harder to make. Effective budget limits would also change the way in which the health care system responds to costly new technologies.

#### Decisions on Resource Allocation

Overall budget limits require someone or some group to decide who gets what kind of care. Within the British hospital this decision is made on a collegial basis by consultants, subject to peer pressure, and by district and regional planning officials, not all of whom are doctors. As we have pointed out earlier, the fact that consultants are salaried and enjoy lifetime tenure purges negotiations among them of personal material considerations. Decisions have personal consequences only as far as the physician's ability to pursue his work is influenced by the availability of beds, staff, and equipment. That concern is obviously important, but removing the issue of income makes the decisionmaking process easier. Our discussions with British physicians and administrators suggest that optimal use of resources in the interests of patient welfare is usually the central focus.

The situation in the United States is quite different. Unlike hospital administrators in Britain, who have little to say about policy, the administrators and the boards of trustees in U.S. hospitals have great power. Although they cannot make day-to-day decisions, they help set policy and also resolve disputes among the medical staff. Given budget limits, they would influence current expenditures as well as both capital outlays and the size and composition of staff, a function carried out largely by higher administrative authorities in Britain.

Under budget limits the importance of hospital administrators would be further heightened because of the incentives to physicians created by the fee-for-service system. In contrast to the British physician, most American doctors have a direct financial stake in decisions that bear on the number of patients they can admit and the diagnostic procedures and treatments they can perform. The desire of physicians to admit and practice as they think best will create conflicts with administrators charged with living under fiscal constraints. The task for physicians and administrators will be to set up procedures under which physicians continue to make day-to-day policy and establish most medical priorities, but administrators make certain that spending priorities are consistent with any guidelines that have been set externally. The existence of spending limits would also encourage the organization of other employee groups in the hospital, most notably nurses, to influence the decision-making process in a way that would protect their interests as well.

### Effects on the Income of Physicians

How the budget constraint is imposed will determine how much the income of the individual physician is affected and thus the amount of intrahospital conflict that will ensue. Diagnostic related groupings are likely to have the least effect, because they do not encourage a reduction in admissions. On the other hand, those physicians who carry out procedures that involve a substantial use of hospital resources are likely to be affected significantly. In the case of overall limits on hospital budgets, cardiac catheterization, angiography, nuclear medicine, and other high-cost diagnostic activities may be reduced in numbers. A limit might also be set on expensive open-heart operations, or the number of operating rooms might be cut in order to restrict surgery. Restrictions might be placed on the number of chronic dialysis patients accepted for treatment or a program like kidney transplantation might be phased out. The physicians responsible for providing such services would, of course, suffer the most financially, but the hospital could then concentrate its resources on areas of special competence or of particular interest to the medical staff. By contrast, procedures such as proctoscopy and bronchoscopy, which involve little in the way of capital equipment or personnel, should be affected least. The overall budget constraint would thus probably produce far more intrahospital conflicts than would limits on reimbursement for defined classes of cases.

### Severity of Limits and Their Effects

In the early stage of trying to slow the growth of hospital expenditures, the stage beyond which no American state has yet moved, limits on expenditures would produce few changes in actual medical practice. Hospitals would be forced to curtail purchases and replacement of equipment, to economize on heating and lighting, to delay replacement of linen, to reduce the quality of food, and to defer maintenance expenditures. Some hospitals would run deficits, rather than the surpluses to which many have been accustomed, and would be forced to dip into endowment funds. Nursing and other staff vacancies would be filled less rapidly than in the past. Workloads would rise and staff morale would fall. Indeed, these effects have been observed under the budget limits now in force in New York.[13]

In the face of only slight constraints, policies regarding admission and treatment would be largely unaffected. Doctors might have to wait a bit longer for lab reports and patients a bit longer to get x-rays than in the days before budget limits. But such important services as surgery and intensive care would be fully staffed. Small changes in quality would occur, such as in the amount of film per x-ray examination, but they would be invisible to patients.

In short, mild budget limits would do little more than subject hospitals to some of the cost discipline that competitive businesses routinely face, but from which hospitals are sheltered by present methods of reimbursement. Mild budget limits on hospitals would squeeze out pure waste and reduce amenities for patients and staff. But savings would be modest.

### Severe Limits, Severe Effects

There is no clear point at which controls on reimbursement of hospitals begin to force decisions that cause substantial reductions in the quality or quantity of some forms of care. If, however, budget constraints became more severe, the days of easy adjustment would end. Decisions would have to be made on what services would be made available to whom. Issues like those faced by Britain would then have to be confronted in the United States. Because the United States would start from a higher expenditure per capita than Britain, the stresses at first would be much less severe and the decisions less draconian. But because public expectations are much higher in the United States than in Britain, the restrictions would be perceived as more painful.

As constraints increased, the effects on patient care would become greater because few options would remain for reducing expenditures without appreciably jeopardizing the patient's welfare. Diagnostic radiology and laboratory examinations are among the most likely choices. As in Britain, hospitals would probably cut back on the number of x-ray examinations as well as on number of films per examination, because the benefits forgone with such reductions are probably small and the potential savings large. Judicious reductions in the number of laboratory tests, nuclear medicine, and other examinations can also be carried out without much loss of useful information. But such cutbacks will not produce savings in proportion to the reduction in tests, for the marginal costs of the procedures, in most instances, are well below the average costs. The introduction of costly new treatments and diagnostic procedures is likely to be slowed until, or even after, effectiveness is clearly demonstrated.

As in Britain, doctors and hospital administrators would be forced to develop rules of thumb for defining what care constitutes standard medical practice and what care is extravagant. Acute illness and traumatic injuries would continue to be diagnosed and treated with the best that each hospital had to offer so long as the victim had even a small chance of recovering and achieving a normal life. Most illnesses of children and young adults would continue to be treated aggressively, much as the British do not stint on the costly treatment of hemophilia. But serious ethical and legal questions would arise in treating the badly impaired and unborn. The treatment of cancer would probably continue to command nearly all the resources required to provide whatever benefit is available. People's fear of cancer would free oncology from the constraints imposed on much of the rest of the system.

Terminal care, on the other hand, would be much reduced. At present, the cost of aggressive care of the terminally ill is borne through increased budgets for health insurance, medicare, medicaid, and other payments by third parties. In short, the price is less consumption of goods and services other than medical care. U.S. practice will probably become more like British practice, where, according to everything we have been told, a lack of intensive care beds and limitations on other specialized technologies preclude aggressive care for dying patients. Such a change will occur because decisions on continuing treatment will be based on considerations far different from present ones. Doctors in the United States realize that aggressive treatment of many terminally ill patients is often pointless, but they cannot do less because of pressure from the patient's family, the fear of malpractice suits, and the threat of intervention by the courts on behalf of the patient.

In a world of resource constraints the rules would inevitably change. The price of continuing to provide such treatment would be death, disability, and pain for nonterminally ill patients denied care because of the use of resources on the terminally ill. Within the present medical system the provision of aggressive care for the terminally ill allows health care providers and the sick person's family to avoid painful personal and professional choices by shifting them to the dry domain of insurance rate-setting and congressional deliberations about government spending; it also allows courts to apply absolutist standards under which the failure to provide care that has any prospect for even small medical benefit is grounds for court intervention or a judgment of malpractice. The problem under budget limits will become like that of triage on the battlefield. The military and its physicians have long understood and accepted the fact that when resources are too few to take care of all the wounded, care is provided to those who stand to benefit the most. The same ethic will apply under the resource limits imposed by budget constraints.

### Limitations on New Therapies

In general, British experience suggests that budget limits would slow the introduction of new therapies and result in lower eventual use than would occur in the absence of constraints. We hypothesize, without evidence from Britain, that therapies in use when the limits go into effect would be less affected than new therapies. It is easier to prevent habits from being formed than it is to break them, and actual commitments evoke a more spirited defense than potential ones. Hospitals would find it easier not to acquire a CT scanner, and still easier not to acquire the technological successor to a CT scanner, than to abandon a CT scanner already installed. Today they would find it far easier not to allow heart transplants, a technology not yet in place, than to tell cardiac surgeons to cut back sharply on coronary artery bypass procedures. Hospitals could more easily put a cap on the use of total parenteral nutrition, by fixing a pharmaceutical budget, than reduce the use of TPN below current levels.

### Total Cost of New Technology

The total cost of a program will also be important in determining whether a new technology is introduced and how widely it is made available. The artificial heart is an excellent example. It has been estimated that some 50,000 people a year would be suitable candidates for this device. Even after the procedure is perfected, the cost is likely to be at least $50,000 a patient and perhaps as much as $100,000 during the first year following surgery, for a total annual expenditure of $2.5 billion to $5 billion. Follow-up costs for the pump that operates the heart, for replacement of malfunctioning hearts, and for general medical care would cause large cumulative additions to the baseline expenditure. Liver, heart, and other transplants would impose similar costs. In an era of commitment to hospital cost containment, society would probably not be willing to make such investments in all medically suitable patients without considering overall costs and whether the beneficiaries of this costly therapy could expect an extended period of high-quality life or a brief extension of life with pain, immobility, and suffering.

### Waiting Lists

Another way to save resources would be by cutting the number of admissions. This could be accomplished in part by reducing discretionary admissions (for example, for vague abdominal pain or mild asthmatic attacks), as is presumably done by HMOs, and in part by allowing waiting lists to develop (for example, for tonsillectomies, cataracts, and hernias). To save much money by those measures, many hospitals would have to close, an outcome that would undoubtedly create political turmoil. Patients value local hospitals and protest not only the threat of closure but even the elimination of certain services.[14] From the self-interest of each community, such a reaction makes sense, particularly because most costs are pooled and borne by payers who may reside elsewhere. Even from the broader standpoint of society, closure may not make sense, because of added transportation costs and delayed treatment.

If waiting lists were allowed to develop, the situation would become even more politically explosive. As in Britain, patients needing elective surgery would be the main group required to wait. But responses in the United States would differ from those in Britain in part because the British have never been accustomed to obtaining all medical care without delay. The National Health Service succeeded a system in which much of the population lacked financial access to health care and had few expectations. Unlike their British counterparts, patients in the United States are accustomed to prompt admission for most procedures and would protest loudly if forced to wait. Physicians would vigorously support their patients' complaints, in part because of personal financial considerations. Fee-for-service reimbursement of physicians would encourage doctors to favor methods of reducing costs other than those that curtail admissions. On the other hand, the high rates of elective surgery in the United States relative to those in Britain[15] suggest that American physicians who now opt for surgery could often recommend nonsurgical treatment without appreciable loss of benefits to the patient.[16]

It is thus hard to imagine lengthy queues for elective surgery in the United States. If no private sector safety valves existed for those who had the means to pay and who would not tolerate delay, either regulations would be relaxed before queues became as long as those in Britain, or other means to conserve resources would be found.

## The Response of Physicians

British experience suggests that budget limits would gradually cause accepted standards of practice to change, even though the incentives of fee-for-service medicine would slow such adjustments. Good medicine would call for fewer tests when the gain in information is slight and for less surgery and less use of costly drugs when the advantage of expensive over inexpensive therapies is small. In short, U.S. doctors would begin to build into their own norms of good practice a sense of the relation between the costs of care and the value of the benefits from it. They would be led to weigh not only the medical aspects of diagnosis and treatment but also the peculiar circumstances of each patient: his age, his underlying health, his family responsibilities, and his chance of recovering enough to resume a normal life.

This process would require a far-reaching change in attitude for the many American doctors who believe it unprofessional, if not immoral, for doctors to consider costs in deciding what actions to take on behalf of patients. One physician summed up this view in a letter to the editor of the *New England Journal of Medicine:*

Optimization of survival and not optimization of cost effectiveness is the only ethical imperative. . . . Ethical physicians do not base their practices on their patient's ability to pay or choose diagnostic or therapeutic procedures on the basis of their cost. . . . Of late an increasing number of articles in this and other journals have been concerned with "cost effectiveness" of diagnostic and therapeutic procedures. Inherent in these articles is the view that choices will be predicated not only on the basis of strictly clinical considerations but also on the basis of economic considerations as they may affect the patient, the hospital and society. It is my contention that such considerations are not germane to ethical medical practice, that they occupy space in journals that would be better occupied by substantive matter, and that they serve to orient physicians toward consideration of economics, which is not their legitimate problem. It is dangerous to introduce extraneous factors into medical decisions, since consideration of such factors may eventually lead to considerations of age, social usefulness, and other matters irrelevant to ethical practice. The example of medicine in Nazi Germany is too close to need further elucidation.[17]

Our observations suggest that, to try to maintain the belief that they are doing everything of value, American physicians, like their British counterparts, will simply redefine what care is "appropriate." Such rationalization is probably essential to the morale of the physician who finds that he must often say no to the patient.

The task of saying no will become increasingly difficult as resource constraints become tighter. British experience indicates, however, that the care most easily denied is that dependent on costly capital goods for its provision. If the authorities do not buy the capital goods—CT scanners, diagnostic x-ray and ultrasound equipment, operating rooms equipped for coronary surgery—the services cannot be provided. If staffing is carefully controlled, doctors, nurses, and other providers are placed in the position of simply doing all they can in the time available. In both cases providers are spared the psychologically insupportable burden of denying care because it is too expensive; rather, they are given the role of allocating existing capacity to the patients who will benefit most from care. In fact, we encountered no instances of capital-intensive activity in which British doctors said that cost dictated care for particular patients. Capacity limits, resulting from earlier decisions on investment and staffing, forced providers to make choices. Because saying no is thus facilitated, we would expect programs that are capital intensive and require large numbers of personnel to be singled out as targets for holding down expenditures.

Services that do not require a specialized capital good or specially trained providers are hard to ration. Aggressive doctors have the opportunity to lay claim to extra resources by incremental steps. The British nephrologist who pushed home dialysis to circumvent limits on hospital-based dialysis was able to greatly increase his command over scarce resources. The doctor who pushed the use of TPN until curbed by his colleagues for draining resources left a legacy of more extensive use of TPN than is common in British hospitals. The aggressive use of new and costly chemotherapeutic drugs to treat cancer in one hospital was stopped only when physicians agreed to subject themselves to a system under which use of these drugs would be monitored.

Controlling expenditures on drugs, blood, and other expendable supplies in the United States will pose one of the most difficult problems in cost containment. Limiting such expenditures by monitoring day-to-day clinical decisions would be almost impossible. Because that mechanism is not practical, a physician could be constrained only if his use of resources was so excessive that, as in Britain, his colleagues forced a change in behavior.

**The Response of Patients**

As budget constraints become tight, patients can be expected to look for safety valves that allow them to obtain care they have been denied. This goal is likely to be pursued far more aggressively in the United States than it has been in Britain because a generation of U.S. patients has come to expect all medical services from which it might benefit.

In Britain, as we have discussed earlier, patients have limited opportunities for working the system to obtain the best possible treatment. Apart from what many British physicians described as the surprising pliability of British patients, the practice of sequential referral, under which the British can see a specialist only if referred by their general practitioner, makes it hard for patients to demand care they are denied. A few patients rebel and present themselves at hospital emergency rooms, although most of that care, as in the United States, is simply primary care provided off-hours when general practitioners are unavailable. The aggressive patient can travel to areas where waiting lists are short, but few are reported to do so.

The opportunity for patients in the United States to fight budget limits would be incomparably greater than it is in Britain. Because patients may visit any physician—general practitioner or specialist—with whom they can secure an appointment, and because the fee-for-service system gives each physician every incentive to accommodate the source of his livelihood, the opportunity for doctor shopping and for cajoling, browbeating, or bribing doctors to provide ''full'' care is magnified. Consequently, aggressive and well-to-do patients would probably obtain superior care and resources would tend to flow toward therapies about which patients are well informed and for which they can recognize the need.

*Getting Care outside the System*

Besides putting more pressure on the physician, patients are likely to try to seek care outside the regulated hospital system. If budget limits are established, a central regulatory and political question will be whether care can be obtained from providers who are not subject to budget limits. A budget limit would have meaning only if some additional cost were imposed on people who chose to purchase services from unregulated providers. How large that additional cost should be is as critical an issue as the level of the budget limit.

The same methods used to control the flow of resources to the mainline hospital system could be used to discourage other providers. These instruments include the tax system, licensing, and limits on reimbursement through public programs or private insurance. Each approach would create a price difference, implicit or explicit, between regulated and unregulated providers.

Each approach would also create political, administrative, and economic problems of its own. In all cases the problems would stem from the desire of people to buy insurance to protect themselves from the risk that a given type of costly care may not be available and from the fact that such insurance inevitably short-circuits the usual incentives of the marketplace to balance costs against benefits.[18]

If these strategies were used to prevent the emergence of providers outside the existing system, the patient might go abroad—for example, to Canada, where the quality of the hospital system is comparable to ours. If enough demand developed, entrepreneurs might open high-quality hospitals in Mexico or the Caribbean. Treatment outside the United States would most often be sought by the affluent, but others might occasionally seek to use this safety valve.

*Charity*

People may wish to escape budget limits for charitable as well as selfish reasons. U.S. hospitals now encourage individual philanthropy and fund-raising drives. The incentives to promote such giving would increase with the restrictiveness of budget limits. As noted in chapter 5, a large proportion of CT scanners in NHS hospitals were donated, and some are run with contributions. British chairs in oncology have been created by private gifts. In one poorly funded district in Britain we were told that charitable gifts provided the only resources to buy many pieces of relatively inexpensive, but important, equipment. Such gifts may be viewed either as an expression of charitable impulses or as a special kind of safety valve permitting individuals or communities to buy medical services that the collectively determined budget is too small to support.

Whatever the motivation or interpretation of such gifts, the authorities must decide whether they violate budget limits and what policy to adopt toward them. If hospitals must operate under an expenditure limit that includes all outlays however financed, charitable contributions would be strongly discouraged, because they would merely supplant payments from other sources and would not increase the hospital's capacity to spend. Alternatively, hospitals might be permitted to treat charitable gifts as additions to their spending ceilings. This approach would provide strong incentives for individuals and businesses to organize fund-raising campaigns if they felt a budget limit was stopping the provision of highly valued services. Indeed, hospitals would probably choose to shortchange precisely those services or facilities around which campaigns for charitable contributions could most easily be organized. Communities, especially the most affluent ones, could circumvent budget limits by organized giving, since charitable contributions are treated even more favorably under the income tax than are medical expenditures.

Gifts of costly capital equipment in the United States might pose the same important problems as in Britain. Acceptance of the gift usually entails a commitment of space and personnel that, over the years, can cost far more than the value of the donation. The British have discovered, moreover, that once funds are raised they are hard to turn down even if they will divert resources from activities that administrators and doctors deem more important. As a result, they sometimes refuse gifts of capital equipment not accompanied by enough funds to cover operating expenses. To avoid this problem, U.S. authorities might choose to limit deductions for charitable contributions to regulated medical providers.

In sum, policies that permit exit from the controlled system and encourage charitable giving will contribute to the adoption and sustainability of fairly tight formal budget limits and will favor those people with high demands for care. Policies that discourage exit and charitable giving will increase the political resistance to budget limits of any given severity, in part because vocal and influential groups will suffer under those policies.

## Litigation

Among the consequences of budget limits, an increase in litigation is the most predictable. The American response will differ strikingly from that of Britain, where, as we have pointed out, few suits are brought because of the restrictions of the British tort system. The claimant in Britain must pay for his lawyer's services regardless of the outcome of the case, and if he loses he is also usually held responsible for the defendant's costs. In contrast, U.S. patients may retain lawyers without out-of-pocket payments. Counsel typically takes one-third of the award if the plaintiff prevails and receives nothing otherwise. Lawyers for the plaintiff can spread their risk over many cases, gains from the winners offsetting any losses. Therefore, even if he is unable to pay an hourly fee, a patient with a seemingly valid complaint can obtain counsel. The contingency fee is thus sometimes described as "the key to the courthouse door."

Because of the characteristics of the U.S. tort system, we anticipate that individual and class action suits would be brought by, and on behalf of, many patients denied some potentially beneficial therapy. Suits would be further stimulated if budget limits prevented physicians from making use of the power to treat fetal defects, to sustain the lives of those whose defects are irremediable, and to carry out procedures that defer or repair the consequences of aging. Doctors would also file suits, alleging financial loss from capricious or erroneous hospital rules.

The issues involved in malpractice claims resulting from budget limits would be complex, and it is not clear how the courts would resolve them. Because hospitals and doctors would choose to cut back different services, therapies unavailable in one place might be obtainable elsewhere. Patients denied a service available at one institution would allege that arbitrary decisions had violated their right to equal protection under the law. Procedures for allocating budgets would be challenged on similar grounds. Ultimately doctors would have to show that their decisions followed standard practice or that decisions to withhold potentially effective care were taken only by carefully observing procedural safeguards. Indeed, the system will largely adapt through a redefinition of the appropriate standard of care under given circumstances.

Judges and juries find it difficult to evaluate a medical dispute, and historically the courts have almost always accepted "customary standards of medical practice" as the standard with which actual behavior is compared.[19] In accepting professional custom as a standard, the legal system considers that physicians as a group, or at least those who set standards, are correctly investing in the avoidance of mishaps and that their judgment can be used as the benchmark of adequate performance. In a world of budget limits, the same legal benchmark will almost certainly be applied.

The redefinition of negligence will obviously be slow. And during the transition period the courts will have no practical way to decide on a day-to-day basis when care should be provided and when it should be withheld. Litigation over the myriad medical decisions appealable under current law would both choke the courts and paralyze medical practice. Thus some procedure would have to be found under which decisions not to give important care were approved by other doctors, and perhaps by lay observers, to avoid the threat of frequent successful legal challenges. Such committees supervised the provision of chronic dialysis in the 1960s before Congress voted to pay for dialysis through medicare. Unfortunately, any such review would seriously and, in some cases, fatally limit the ability of doctors to make quick decisions. Even if the procedure worked fast enough, the demise of clinical freedom would convert many medical decisions from individual to committee actions. Any mode of resolution would lead to controversy.

### Political Pressure

Some dissatisfied patients will appeal to their elected representatives. Congressional mail will abound with horror stories describing how a sick relative is being denied dialysis, bone marrow transplantation, hip replacement, or some other potentially beneficial procedure. To satisfy the constituent, congressional staff is likely to bring pressure on the hospital or at least to make an inquiry to see that a fair decision has been made. Executive agencies of federal and state governments might respond similarly. All this will add to administrative complexity.

Parents and families will also turn to the media, which, recognizing the wide appeal of heart-rending stories, will highlight the effects of the budget shortfall. Constituent pressure could become so widespread and intense that Congress might begin to mandate specific exceptions to the budget constraints. Chronic dialysis, heart, liver, and other organ transplants, or artificial skin could be excluded from the limits, and the system of control would then slowly become more porous. If such pressure should prevail, it would suggest that the public or a vocal minority wants more investment in health care than the limited budget permits.

These pressures are not hypothetical. Already in 1983 the plight of infants requiring liver transplants for survival had become the subject of congressional hearings. Evening news programs beamed nationwide the image of wan children whose lives were reported to hinge on access to costly surgery. Similar responses to new and expensive technologies seem inevitable.


### Conclusions

To avoid forcing people to weigh costs and benefits at the time of illness and to prevent expensive treatment from becoming financially catastrophic for individuals and their families, all developed nations have devised institutions to insulate patients from the cost of care at the time that it is needed. These institutions differ from country to country, but their effect is the same: to encourage patients to seek all potentially beneficial care and the doctors to provide it. When technology supplied few diagnostic or therapeutic techniques that promised mitigation or cure of disease, the cost of such protection was not great.

Since World War II the picture has changed dramatically. Modern medicine possesses a large and growing armory of increasingly costly weapons for dealing with illness. They may produce large benefits in some cases, but in many others benefits are small relative to the cost of providing them. The dilemma that the United States and many other rich nations face is how to encourage patients and providers to weigh in a humane fashion the benefits and costs of medical care. Most such nations have laboriously created institutions that shield patients from out-of-pocket medical costs. Yet these very institutions, in association with technological change, are largely responsible for creating the problem of rising costs that many nations now seek to solve. The British have minimized this problem by the simple expedient of a budget limit. Whether budgets have been set too high or too low is a matter on which disagreement is certain and legitimate. Whether available budgets have been allocated to the services with the highest possible benefits is also open to dispute.

We are persuaded that the United States is not interested in creating a national health service on the British model. Without such direct collective control over the allocation of resources to health care, the United States must rely on other means.

The federal government has tried to hold down costs by limiting purchases of equipment and controlling the number of hospital beds. These programs have enjoyed few successes. Several states have begun to experiment with programs to limit hospital budgets, chiefly by mandatory prospective reimbursement; these efforts appear to be more promising. Successive presidents have proposed federal limits on hospital spending. But except for temporary controls as an element of general price controls under President Nixon, no proposal was adopted until the 1982 legislation that mandated fixed reimbursement for medicare patients according to diagnostic related groupings.

We expect that in the future various methods of trying to slow the growth of hospital expenditures will be tried. If they become effective, the United States will have to confront the range of problems described in this book. The fundamental conflict between a fee-for-service system of reimbursing physicians and efforts to limit hospital expenditures will emerge. Policies will have to be developed on safety valves, on malpractice suits, and on the introduction of new technologies—policies that current ways of providing hospital care make unnecessary.

We cannot know how vigorous will be American attempts to hold down hospital spending. Many forces will be arrayed against the implementation and enforcement of limits that force rationing of care, that cut into incomes of doctors, nurses, and other staff, or that significantly curtail sales by hospital suppliers. The history of efforts to regulate industry in the United States is littered with cases in which the industry subject to regulation gained control of the agency to which it was legally subject.

The choices we face are clear and painful. The United States can suffer a continual increase in medical expenditures and in expenditures yielding benefits worth less than costs. Or it can impose effective limits. If it follows the second course, it will have to confront a long list of hard decisions on which discussion has not yet begun. Rationing will inevitably be a painful prescription.

*appendix* **Hip Replacement**

The statement in chapter 4 that the British do three-fourths to four-fifths as many hip replacements as the Americans summarizes the results of five different estimates. The main problem is that sources of data from Britain are not explicit in defining what procedures are included in various statistics.

**U.S. Data**

The National Center for Health Statistics collects data on the frequency of various surgical procedures. Donald Smith of NCHS supplied us with data on the number and age of patients who underwent hip surgery in 1979. The data are broken down under two headings: total hip replacement (including "total hip replacement with use of methyl methacrylate" and "other total hip replacement") and other arthroplasty of the hip (including "replacement of head of femur with use of methyl methacrylate," "other replacement of head of femur," "replacement of acetabulum with use of methyl methacrylate," "other replacement of acetabulum," and "other repair of hip").

In 1979, 130,367 people received hip surgery of all kinds, including 59,927 hip replacements. Some people, however, were operated on more than once. No data exist on exactly how many such people there were, but Melton and others report that the number of total hip-joint replacements in 1980 was 58,000 or 59,000 but that the total number of separate procedures may have been closer to 70,000.[1]

**British Data**

British data are contained in Department of Health and Social Security, *Orthopaedic Services: Waiting Time for Out-Patient Appointments and In-Patient Treatment* (London: Her Majesty's Stationery Office, 1981). This source reports that in 1977 about 37,290 operations were performed for arthroplasty of the hip, about 27,080 operations for arthroplasty of the hip in connection with osteoarthritis or a fracture of the neck of the femur, and about 14,200 of those for arthroplasty of the hip "which relates to osteoarthritis, namely total joint replacement."

### Method of Comparison

We computed the rate per million of population in each country that underwent surgery under each of these five definitions (two for the United States, three for England and Wales). Then we used the population of the other country to calculate how many operations would be performed if that rate of surgery prevailed. In making these comparisons, we assumed that the broadest of the three definitions for England and Wales (according to which 37,290 hip operations were performed in 1977) corresponds to the broader definition for the United States (according to which 130,367 people underwent surgery). We arbitrarily increased the statistics for the United States to 145,000 to take into account that some U.S. patients had more than one hip operated on. We assumed that the narrowest definition from England and Wales corresponds to the narrower definition for the United States.

Using population statistics from U.S. Bureau of the Census, *Statistical Abstract of the United States, 1979* (Government Printing Office, 1979), pp. 29, 32; and Central Statistical Office, *Annual Abstract of Statistics, 1980* (HMSO, 1980), p. 15, we reached the following estimates. If one concentrates on the narrower definitions in each country, the rate of total hip replacement in England and Wales is 74 to 77 percent of that in the United States, depending on which population weights are used. If one focuses on the broadest definition, the rate of all hip surgery in England and Wales is about as high as that in the United States. Thus Britain seems to be doing more operations short of total hip replacement than does the United States, quite possibly in connection with broken hips of elderly women, a type of surgery that according to many reports is leading to "blocked beds" in British hospitals.

# Notes

## Chapter 1 (pages 3–11)

1. Hospital care expenditures alone showed even more dramatic increases, rising from $153 per capita in 1950, to $257 in 1965, and to $563 in 1981. Robert M. Gibson and Daniel R. Waldo, "National Health Expenditures, 1981," *Health Care Financing Review*, vol. 4 (September 1982), pp. 19–21. We used a medical care deflator to calculate expenditures in 1982 dollars. *Economic Report of the President, January 1983*, p. 221.

2. For details on these controls, see Paul B. Ginsberg, "Inflation and the Economic Stabilization Program," in Michael Zubkoff, ed., *Health: A Victim or a Cause of Inflation?* (New York: Prodist for the Milbank Memorial Fund, 1976), pp. 31–51.

3. *The Budget of the United States Government, Fiscal Year 1978*, p. 159.

4. Congressional Budget Office, *The Hospital Cost Containment Act of 1977: An Analysis of the Administration's Proposal*, prepared for the Subcommittee on Health and Scientific Research of the Senate Committee on Human Resources, 95 Cong. 1 sess. (Government Printing Office, 1977), p. 6.

5. David S. Salkever and Thomas W. Bice, *Hospital Certificate-of-Need Controls: Impact on Investment, Costs, and Use* (Washington, D.C.: American Enterprise Institute for Public Policy Research, 1979), p. 75; William B. Schwartz, "The Regulation Strategy for Controlling Hospital Costs," *New England Journal of Medicine*, vol. 305 (November 19, 1981), pp. 1249–55; Frank A. Sloan, *Insurance, Regulation and Hospital Costs* (Lexington Books, 1980), pp. 94, 96, 171–73; and William B. Schwartz and Paul L. Joskow, "Duplicated Hospital Facilities: How Much Can We Save by Consolidating Them?" *New England Journal of Medicine*, vol. 303 (December 18, 1980), pp. 1449–57.

6. Craig Coelen and Daniel Sullivan, "An Analysis of the Effects of Prospective Reimbursement Programs on Hospital Expenditures," *Health Care Financing Review*, vol. 2 (Winter 1981), pp. 1–40; Frank Sloan, "Regulation and the Rising Cost of Hospital Care," *Review of Economics and Statistics*, vol. 63 (November 1981), pp. 479–87; and Schwartz, "Regulation Strategy for Controlling Hospital Costs."

7. Congressional Budget Office, *Controlling Rising Hospital Costs* (GPO, 1979), p. 60. Not all programs are effective, at least during their first years. New Jersey's use of diagnostic related groupings (fixed reimbursements for carefully defined procedures) to control hospital costs is reported not to have initially decreased expenditures. John K. Iglehart, "Health Policy Report: New Jersey's Experiment with DRG-Based Hospital Reimbursement," *New England Journal of Medicine*, vol. 307 (December 23, 1982), pp. 1655–60.

8. "A New System for Hospital Payment: The Massachusetts Plan," *National Journal*, vol. 14 (August 21, 1982), pp. 1488–89; Jean Dietz, "Hospital Chiefs Draft Cuts under New Cost Control Law," *Boston Globe*, September 30, 1982; Richard A.

Knox, "How Hospital Law Will Work," *Boston Globe,* August 24, 1982; Liz Roman Gallese, "Massachusetts Law Offers New Approach to Cut Hospital Costs," *Wall Street Journal,* August 13, 1982; Massachusetts Hospital Association, "Proposal for a Prospective Reimbursement System Demonstration for Medicare," revised (Boston, August 1982); and Brian Biles and others, "Hospital Cost Inflation under State Rate-Setting Programs," *New England Journal of Medicine,* vol. 303 (September 18, 1980), p. 666.

9. We do not describe the American health care system for British readers. An excellent brief summary of the American and Canadian health care systems, together with comparative data on those two systems and that of Britain, is found in Jeremy Hurst, "Financing Health Services in the United States, Canada, and Britain," Nuffield/Leveshulme Fellowship Report (London, November 1982).

**Chapter 2 (pages 12–25)**

1. The United Kingdom spent 5.3 percent of its gross national product on health care in 1980; the United States spent 9.4 percent. The British per capita gross domestic product (GDP) in 1980 was 61 percent of the American figure, according to forecasts of relative per capita GDP in the international consensus of real gross product. Daniel R. Waldo and Robert M. Gibson, "National Health Expenditures, 1980," *Health Care Financing Review,* vol. 3 (September 1981), p. 18; International Monetary Fund, *International Financial Statistics Yearbook, 1981,* vol. 34 (IMF, 1981), pp. 437–41; "At Home and Abroad," *Lancet,* vol. 1 (January 2, 1982), p. 24; and Irving B. Kravis and others, *World Product and Income: International Comparisons of Real Gross Product* (Johns Hopkins University Press, 1982), p. 16.

2. Without any adjustments, the United States spent $850 per capita on health care in 1978, while Britain spent $306. Jeremy Hurst, "An Aggregate Comparison of the Performance of the American and British Health Sectors" (U.K. Department of Health and Social Security, 1981), table C1. If the U.S. figure is deflated by subtracting the relative wage superiority of American doctors, other pay advantages in the United States, and the pay advantage of other hospital personnel, and if costs for administration, research, and construction are subtracted from both sides, the adjusted totals for hospital expenditures are $327.33 per capita in the United States and $173.96 per capita in Britain. See table 6-1 in this volume.

3. Hospital bed data: American Hospital Association, *Hospital Statistics, 1981,* p. 3; and U.K. Department of Health and Social Security, *Health and Personal Social Services Statistics for England, 1978* (London: Her Majesty's Stationery Office, 1978), p. 73. Physician data: U.S. Department of Health and Human Services, Office of Health Research, Statistics, and Technology, *Health United States, 1981* (HHS, 1981), p. 177; and DHSS, *Health and Personal Social Services Statistics, 1978,* pp. 36, 54, 70. Nurse data: U.S. Bureau of the Census, *Statistical Abstract of the United States, 1981* (Government Printing Office, 1981), p. 104; and DHSS, *Health and Personal Social Services Statistics, 1978,* p. 28. Admissions data: AHA, *Hospital Statistics, 1981,* p. 3; and DHSS, *Health and Personal Social Services Statistics, 1978,* p. 74.

4. Bureau of the Census, *Statistical Abstract of the United States, 1981,* pp. 69–73; HHS, National Center for Health Statistics, *Advance Report of Final Mortality Statistics, 1979,* supplement of *Monthly Vital Statistics Report,* vol. 31, no. 6 (1982); DHSS, *Health and Personal Social Services Statistics for England, 1982* (HMSO, 1982); and Central Statistical Office, *Annual Abstract of Statistics, 1983* (HMSO, 1983), p. 40.

5. A. J. Culyer, *The British Health Service: An Economic Perspective* (University of York, 1978), p. 20; and British Information Services, *Health Services in Britain* (London: Unwin, 1977), p. 4.

6. Economic Models Limited, *The British Health Care System* (American Medical Association, 1976), pp. 31, 35; and Culyer, *British Health Service,* pp. 20–21.

7. Culyer, *British Health Service,* p. 23; Gwyn Bevan and others, *Health Care Priorities and Management* (London: Croom Helm, 1980), p. 281; Jeremy Hurst, "Financing Health Services in the United States, Canada, and Britain," Nuffield/Levershulme Fellowship Report (London, November 1982), pp. 66, 68; *Royal Commission on the National Health Service Report* (HMSO, 1979), p. 431; and International Monetary Fund, *International Financial Statistics Yearbook, 1980,* p. 429.

8. Anthony J. Culyer, *Need and the National Health Service* (Totowa, N.J.: Rowman and Littlefield, 1976), p. 115; Peter Townsend, "Inequality and the Health Service," *Lancet,* vol. 1 (June 15, 1974), pp. 1179–90; John Goodman, *Health Care in Great Britain: Lessons for the U.S.A.* (Fisher Institute, 1980), pp. 75–84, 175–82; William H. Stewart and Philip E. Enterline, "Effects of the National Health Service on Physician Utilization and Health in England and Wales," *New England Journal of Medicine,* vol. 265 (December 14, 1961), pp. 1187–94; Mary-Ann Rozbicki, "Rationing British Health Care: The Cost/Benefit Approach," U.S. Department of State, Executive Seminar in National and International Affairs, Twentieth Session (GPO, 1978), p. 15; J. Rogers Hollingsworth, "Inequality in Levels of Health in England and Wales, 1891–1971," Discussion Paper 581-79 (University of Wisconsin–Madison, Institute for Research on Poverty, November 1979), pp. 16–27; and Peter D. Fox, "Managing Health Resources: English Style," in Gordon McLachlin, ed., *By Guess or by What? Information without Design in the NHS* (Oxford: Oxford University Press, 1978), p. 3.

9. DHSS, *Health and Personal Social Services Statistics for England, 1982,* pp. 51, 104; and Fox, "Managing Health Resources," pp. 11, 14.

10. The report of a Working Party on Orthopedic Services states that in 1979, 73 percent of urgent cases awaiting surgery had waited more than one month and 33 percent of all nonurgent cases had waited more than one year. DHSS, *Orthopaedic Services: Waiting Time for Out-Patient Appointments and In-Patient Treatment* (HMSO, 1981), p. 5.

11. *British Medical Journal,* vol. 285 (November 6, 1982), p. 1363; and *Royal Commission Report,* p. 126.

12. See R. R. West and B. McKibbin, "Shortening Waiting Lists in Orthopedic Surgery Outpatient Clinics," *British Medical Journal,* vol. 284 (March 6, 1982), pp. 728–30.

13. DHSS, *Orthopaedic Services,* p. 6. One problem is that the meaning of waiting lists depends in part on whether all patients are eventually admitted, and on whether waiting times are rising or falling.

14. DHSS, *Health and Personal Social Services Statistics for England, 1977* (HMSO, 1977), p. 21; British Information Services, *Health Services in Britain* (BIS, 1977), p. 9; and Hurst, "Financing Health Services," p. 41.

15. Fox, "Managing Health Resources," pp. 14–15; and "A Cash Limit on Family Practitioner Services," *Lancet,* vol. 2 (August 8, 1981), pp. 317–18.

16. Hurst, "Financing Health Services," pp. 7, 44.

17. Bevan and others, *Health Care Priorities,* pp. 75–79.

18. Ibid., p. 79.

19. From 1976 to 1982 adjustments were made in the budgets for the succeeding year; before 1976 adjustments were made during the current year. Ibid., pp. 76–79, and correspondence with Jeremy Hurst.

20. Bevan and others, *Health Care Priorities,* pp. 143–45. The adjustment includes flows of *inpatients* across boundaries, but not of day or outpatient services. Regression analysis is used to estimate the average costs of treatment. But in light of econometric problems and notoriously inaccurate data, one must view the adjustment skeptically.

21. Information was supplied in a letter from B. E. Godfrey, August 15, 1980.

22. DHSS, "Whole Body Scanners in England and Wales," n.d., p. 1.

23. *Nominal* equality in Britain translates into real *inequality* because the cost of living differs among regions. Such differences in real wages probably help reduce inequality in the distribution of medical personnel by providing a real wage bonus to providers who choose to locate in poorly served areas with low living costs. See William B. Schwartz and others, "The Changing Geographic Distribution of Board-Certified Physicians," *New England Journal of Medicine,* vol. 303 (October 30, 1980), pp. 1032–38.

24. DHSS, *The Way Forward—Priorities in the Health and Social Services* (HMSO, 1977), p. 7.

25. Medical need, in turn, was population-weighted for specific services. The need for nonpsychiatric inpatient services was determined by the "population weighted by national bed utilization rates for age, sex, and condition and adjusted by the standardized fertility ratio . . . and by the standardized mortality ratio." Alan Maynard and Anne Ludbrook, "Budget Allocation in the National Health Service," *Journal of Social Policy,* vol. 9 (July 1980), pp. 289–312.

26. DHSS, *Sharing Resources for Health in England,* Report of the Resource Allocation Working Party (HMSO, 1976), pp. 30–33; DHSS, *Priorities for Health and Personal Social Services in England* (HMSO, 1976), p. 1; "The Honeymoon Is Over," *Health and Social Service Journal,* March 7, 1980, p. 320; and Rodney Deitch, "Has the Government Given Up the NHS?" *Lancet,* vol. 1 (March 20, 1982), p. 693.

27. Whatever procedure they use, authorities in each region allocate budgets to the districts within them. Not all the resources provided to each district are distributed in this way. Some funds are retained for direct purchases by the regions, and some allocations to the districts are made to cover services or facilities that are intended to serve the entire region and, on occasion, other regions as well. For example, a region may have one or two CT scanners or one or two centers for cardiac surgery, and the blood fractionation laboratory at Oxford serves the whole country. In the budget there is, however, a crude recognition that the districts in which CT scanners or other scarce facilities are located must serve the entire region.

28. "Pay Beds," *British Medical Journal,* vol. 285 (November 6, 1982), p. 1364.

29. "Private Hospital Beds," *British Medical Journal,* vol. 284 (February 13, 1982); information supplied in a letter from Jeremy Hurst; and Lee Donaldson Associates, *U.K. Private Medical Care: Provident Schemes Statistics, 1980* (London: Pereguine, 1981), table 10.

30. Compared with users of the NHS, private patients spend proportionately more on drugs than on any other type of medical care. Therefore, the ratio of private outlays to total medical expenditures (which include drug costs) is higher than the ratio of private outlays to total expenditures on physicians and inpatient care. (Information was supplied in a letter from Jeremy Hurst, August 1980.)

31. *Royal Commission Report,* pp. 285–86.

32. The proportion of consultants with some type of private practice ranges from 63 to 71 percent in the London area and from 18 to 58 percent elsewhere in Great Britain. Ibid., app. E, p. 430.

33. Economic Models Limited, *British Health Care System,* p. 147.

34. Lee Donaldson Associates, *U.K. Private Medical Care*, p. 4.

35. Jonathan Spivak, "Private Health Care in Britain," *Wall Street Journal*, August 21, 1979.

36. Jeremy W. Hurst, "Financing Health Services," pp. 78–81.

37. Michael Lee, *Private and National Health Services* (Policy Studies Institute, 1978), pp. 21–22.

38. The low occupancy rates resulted partly from the superior amenities available for minor procedures in privately owned facilities and the hostility of some NHS hospital employees toward private patients, partly from shortened average stays, and partly from increased charges. *Royal Commission Report*, p. 291; and Lee, *Private and National Health Services*, p. 12.

## Chapter 3 (pages 29–56)

1. G. Pincherle, *Topics of Our Time, 2: Kidney Transplants and Dialysis* (London: Her Majesty's Stationery Office, 1979), p. 25.

2. H. Krakauer and others, "The Recent U.S. Experience in the Treatment of End-Stage Renal Disease by Dialysis and Transplantation," *New England Journal of Medicine*, vol. 308 (June 30, 1983), pp. 1558–63. Most fatalities are due to heart disease, stroke, and infections. Lawrence E. Earley and Carl W. Gottschalk, eds., *Strauss and Welt's Diseases of the Kidney*, 3d ed. (Little, Brown, 1979), pp. 421–62.

3. Krakauer and others, "Recent U.S. Experience."

4. Asad A. Bakir and George Dunea, "Current Trends in the Treatment of Uraemia: A View from the United States," *British Medical Journal*, vol. 1 (April 7, 1979), p. 915; Office of Health Economics, *Renal Failure: A Priority in Health?* (London: OHE, 1978), pp. 42–43; Pincherle, *Topics of Our Time, 2*, p. 16; and Gordon Scorer and Anthony Wing, eds., *Decision Making in Medicine: The Practice of Its Ethics* (London: Edward Arnold, 1979), p. 161.

5. These figures probably do not take into account all the economic costs of home dialysis, such as necessary home remodeling and, more important, the services provided by other family members. Proper imputation for such costs might not eliminate, but would certainly narrow, the differences. In contrast, estimates of the cost of center dialysis do not include the cost to the patient of fitting his schedule to the demands of a commercial enterprise. Whether it is more cost-effective to dialyze a patient in the home or in a center depends more on the social considerations of the mode of treatment and on the preferences of the patient and his or her family—that is, on effectiveness—than on cost, if by cost one includes all relevant economic costs. Philip J. Held and Mark V. Pauly, "Competition and Efficiency in the End Stage Renal Disease Program," *Journal of Health Economics*, vol. 2 (August 1983), pp. 95–118.

6. "Kidney Failure," *British Medical Journal*, vol. 284 (March 13, 1982), p. 834; and Pincherle, *Topics of Our Time, 2*, p. 6.

7. *Combined Report on Regular Dialysis and Transplantation in Europe, XI, 1980*, (Basel: Hospal, Ltd., 1980), p. 3; Scorer and Wing, eds., *Decision Making in Medicine*, p. 162; Health Care Financing Administration, "End-Stage Renal Disease Program Highlights, 1982" (HCFA, 1983); and Henry Krakauer and others, "Medical and Fiscal Impact of Alternative Strategies for End-Stage Renal Disease" (National Institute of Allergy and Infectious Diseases, 1983).

8. Scorer and Wing, eds., *Decision Making in Medicine*, p. 162.

9. V. Parsons and P. Lock, "Triage and the Patient with Renal Failure," *Journal of Medical Ethics,* vol. 6 (December 1980), pp. 173–76; and Medical Services Study Group of the Royal College of Physicians, "Deaths from Chronic Renal Failure under the Age of 50," *British Medical Journal,* vol. 283 (July 25, 1981), pp. 283–86.

10. "Ethics and the Nephrologist," *Lancet,* vol. 1 (March 14, 1981).

11. Letter from Professor Oliver M. Wrong, School of Medicine, University College, London, July 7, 1982. See also "Ethics and the Nephrologist," and Report of the Executive Committee of the Renal Association, "Distribution of Nephrological Services for Adults in Great Britain," *British Medical Journal,* vol. 2 (October 16, 1976), pp. 903–06.

12. Medical Services Study Group, "Deaths from Chronic Renal Failure"; and "Audit in Renal Failure: The Wrong Target?" *British Medical Journal,* vol. 283 (July 25, 1981), pp. 261–62, 555–57.

13. Office of Health Economics, *End Stage Renal Failure* (London: White Crescent Press, 1980), pp. 1–8.

14. Severe hemophiliacs have less than 1 or 2 percent of the normal amount of the deficient factor and will suffer an average of forty hemorrhages a year. Moderate hemophiliacs have up to 5 or 10 percent of the deficient factor and will suffer an average of fifteen hemorrhages a year. Mild hemophiliacs have more than 5 or 10 percent of the deficient factor and will suffer an average of two episodes a year. U.S. Department of Health, Education, and Welfare, National Institutes of Health, *Study to Evaluate the Supply-Demand Relationships for AHF and PTC through 1980* (HEW, 1977), pp. 6, 16, 21; Rosemary Biggs and J. D. Spolr, "National Survey of Haemophilia and Christmas Disease Patients in the United Kingdom," *Lancet,* vol. 1 (May 27, 1978), pp. 1143–44; National Institutes of Health, *Summary Report: NHLI's Blood Resource Studies, June 30, 1972* (HEW, 1973), p. 108; and Rosemary Biggs, "Haemophilia Treatment in the United Kingdom from 1969 to 1974," *British Journal of Haematology,* vol. 35 (1977), pp. 489, 491.

15. M. L. Stirling and R. J. Prescott, "Minimum Effective Dose of Intermediate Factor VIII Concentrate in Haemophiliacs on Home Therapy," *Lancet,* vol. 1 (April 14, 1979), p. 814; discussion with Dr. Peter Jones, June 5, 1980; Peter H. Levine, "Hemophilia and Allied Conditions," in Howard L. Cown, ed., *Current Therapy* (W. B. Saunders, 1979), p. 271; John Stuart and others, "Improving Prospects for Employment of the Haemophiliac," *British Medical Journal,* vol. 280 (May 10, 1980), p. 1169; Felicity Carter and others, "Cost of Management of Patients with Haemophilia," *British Medical Journal,* vol. 2 (August 1976), p. 466; Louis Aledort, "Lessons from Hemophilia," *New England Journal of Medicine,* vol. 306 (March 11, 1982), p. 607; and Peter Jones, ed., *Haemophilia Home Therapy* (London: Pitman Medical, 1980), p. 131.

16. Information on the trend toward prophylaxis is based on correspondence with Dr. Peter Jones, September 9, 1981; letter from Diana Walford, May 12, 1980; and National Institutes of Health, *Study to Evaluate the Supply-Demand Relationships,* exhibit III.

17. Stirling and Prescott, "Minimum Effective Dose of Intermediate Factor VIII," p. 813; Richard I. Harris and John Stuart, "Low-Dose Factor VIII in Adults with Haemophilic Arthropathy," *Lancet,* vol. 1 (January 13, 1979), p. 93; A. Aronstam and others, "Double-Blind Controlled Trial of Three Dosage Regimen in Treatment of Haemarthroses in Haemophilia A," *Lancet,* vol. 1 (January 26, 1980), p. 169; and Peter Jones, ed., *Haemophilia Home Therapy,* p. 111.

18. The U.S. figures exclude carcinoma in situ and nonmelanoma skin cancers. The

incidence of cancer and death from cancer is thus appreciably higher in Britain. The death rate in the United States is approximately 1,800 per million annually and in Britain about 2,500 per million. The British figure is based on a total number of cancer cases in the United Kingdom of about 400,000 and the estimate that skin cancer and carcinoma of the uterine cervix in situ amounted to 30 to 40 percent of the total. The resulting estimate of 235,000 cases is about twice as large as the 114,000 cases treated with radiotherapy. The ratio in the United States is similar (353,000 cases treated versus 700,000 total). American Cancer Society, *Cancer Facts and Figures, 1979* (New York: ACS, 1979), p. 10; National Center for Health Statistics, *Advance Report of Final Mortality Statistics, 1979*, supplement of *Monthly Vital Statistics Report*, vol. 31, no. 6 (1982); and Government Statistical Service, *Annual Abstract of Statistics, 1980* (HMSO, 1980).

19. Update of Cancer Patient Survival Statistics (December 1982), prepared by the National Cancer Institute, Vincent T. DeVita, Jr., M.D., director.

20. The number of cases treated with megavoltage units was 350,028, according to the Radiation Therapy Oncology Group, *Patterns of Care Study Survey* (Philadelphia: American College of Radiology, 1977). The guidelines are from William B. Schwartz and Paul L. Joskow, "Duplicated Hospital Facilities: How Much Can We Save by Consolidating Them?" *New England Journal of Medicine*, vol. 303 (December 18, 1980), pp. 1449–57.

21. Britain has 164 megavolt machines. Data are from "Hospital Physicists Association Survey," provided by Dr. Ronald Oliver of the Department of Health and Social Services in letter dated March 12, 1982. The corresponding data for the United States are 1,504 machines. Simon Kramer and others, "Summary Results from the Facilities Master List Survey Conducted by the Patterns of Care Study Group," *International Journal of Radiation Oncology, Biology, and Physics*, no. 8 (1982), table 6.

22. The figure of 117,000 for number of patients receiving radiotherapy is taken from DHSS, *Health and Personal Social Services Statistics for England, 1978* (HMSO, 1978), p. 80. The estimate of the percent treated for skin cancer is based on the South Thames Registry, 1975. The calculation was carried out in the following way: the total number of patients receiving radiotherapy in South Thames was 31 percent of the total cancer group, or 7,779. Of the 2,843 skin patients in the registry, 51 percent, or 1,449, received radiotherapy. Thus 1,449/7,779, or 19 percent, received radiotherapy. This number agrees closely with the value of 22 percent for number of skin cancers among patients treated by the Radiotherapy Service in Cardiff, Wales. Memorandum from Professor Thomas J. Deeley, director of the Radiotherapy Center at the Velindre Hospital, September 22, 1982. The British figure compares with the 1,604 per million receiving radiotherapy annually in the United States for cancers other than cancer of the skin or cancer in situ; that is, 350,028 cases treated in a population of 220 million. The figure of sixteen treatments per patient is based on Radiation Therapy Staff Working Group, *Radiation Therapy in Massachusetts: Resource Inventory and Utilization* (Office of State Health Planning, Massachusetts Department of Public Health, 1979), p. 14. In the United Kingdom a linear accelerator can be used to treat fifty to sixty patients a day. R. F. Mould, "Radiotherapy Treatment Workload Statistics," *Physics in Medicine and Biology*, vol. 27 (January 1982), pp. 157–62. Assuming 250 days a year of operation, this would mean a load of 12,500 to 15,000 treatments a year.

23. Memorandum from Professor Thomas J. Deeley, September 22, 1982. According to Deeley, palliative treatment in the United Kingdom usually consists of one, two, or three treatments and radical (curative) courses involve twenty treatments or less. Because about half the patients receive palliative treatment, the average number of

courses per patient across the group as a whole is apparently well below sixteen. The British also have seventy-seven units of 300 kilovolt capacity (see "Hospital Physicists Association Survey"). About half the patients requiring radiotherapy need palliation only, and about one-third of these have symptoms that can be relieved with less than megavoltage treatment. In the United Kingdom, therefore, about 17,000 of the 92,000 patients who require radiotherapy could be handled with 300-kilovolt machines. Such treatment is, of course, less than optimal because of the resulting skin injury.

24. The radiotherapist is a physician (often in charge of the radiation department) who is responsible for planning therapy. The physicist ensures radiation safety, makes equipment choices, and provides technical planning of dosage. The mechanics of setting up the machine and the patient are the responsibility of the radiotherapy technician.

25. In 1977 less than 5 percent of the units in the United Kingdom fell into the category of greater than 10 MeV, while in the United States the number was 11 percent. Kramer and others, "Summary Results," table 6; and S. Jeffrey, "Radiotherapy Equipment (1977): Major Centres with Megavoltage Equipment" (DHSS, n.d.). The lifetime cost of cobalt 60 units and linear accelerators in the 4 to 6 MeV range is about the same. The linear accelerator costs $400,000 to $500,000. The cobalt unit costs $200,000, but its energy source must be replaced every three years, so that over the usual decade or more of use the cost is similar to that of the accelerator. To the cost of either machine must be added the price of installation (shielding and weight-bearing floor), which adds another $100,000 or so to bring the total expenditure to $500,000–$600,000. Communication from Dr. Edward Sternick, director, Medical Physics Division, Department of Therapeutic Radiology, New England Medical Center, April 20, 1982. The initial cost for high-energy accelerators is $900,000 to $1,800,000, and with an installation cost of $200,000 the overall cost will approach or exceed $1,000,000, two to four times that of the lower-energy instruments. The betatron, which is rated at 20 to 45 MeV, is equally expensive, costing over $2 million with installation. Communication from Dr. Edward Sternick, April 20, 1982.

26. Discussion with Dr. Hywel Madoc-Jones, chief, Department of Therapeutic Radiology, New England Medical Center, October 6, 1981.

27. American radiotherapists disagree about the relative merits of cobalt 60 units and the usual 4 to 6 MeV linear accelerator. Some believe that the linear accelerator offers appreciable advantages, where others believe that any difference between the two is trivial. (This statement is based on discussions with Dr. Hywel Madoc-Jones and with Dr. Anthony Piro, chief of radiotherapy, Salem Hospital, October 1981.) But this issue need not be examined here, because cobalt 60 units represent about 60 percent of the total units in each country. Some 16 percent of cobalt 60 machines in the United States and 18 percent in the United Kingdom are more than fifteen years old. See "Hospital Physicists Association Survey," and letter from Dr. James J. Diamond, Radiation Oncology Study Group, American College of Radiology, October 21, 1981.

28. Recommendation on proportion of radiotherapists from Committee for Radiation Oncology Studies, *Criteria for Radiation Oncology in Multidisciplinary Cancer Management*, Report to the Director of the National Cancer Institute, National Institutes of Health (NIH, 1981). In the United States about 2,000 full-time-equivalent radiotherapists care for a population of 353,000 patients a year, or about one radiotherapist for 177 patients. Letter from Dr. James Diamond, October 21, 1981. In the United Kingdom about 330 full-time-equivalent radiotherapists care for an estimated 95,000 patients a year, or one radiotherapist for 288 patients. DHSS, *Health and Personal Social Services Statistics for England, 1978*, p. 39.

29. Letter from Dr. Anthony Piro, chief of radiotherapy, Salem Hospital.

30. The British have 164 megavoltage machines, which require at least 328 technologists, and 171 low-voltage units, which require 171 technologists. Letter from Ronald Oliver of DHSS. If one assumes that they have one simulator for every two megavoltage units, an additional 82 technologists would be needed for a total of 581. They actually have 736. If one assumes that they have three technologists per megavoltage unit, the ratio most recommended, the number would rise to 738, a value almost identical to that which they report. This latter value seems credible because a slight shortage of radiotherapists can be made up, perhaps at a small loss of quality, by a favorable pattern of staffing by technicians. *A Proposal for Integrated Cancer Management in the United States: The Role of Radiation Oncology,* Report to the National Cancer Institute, National Institutes of Health (NIH, 1972), p. 8. From a sample consisting of 90 percent of U.S. facilities, there appear to be 2,955 full-time-equivalent radiotherapy technologists. This number is four times as large as in Britain, just as the population of the United States and the cancer patient load is presumably four times as large. But because the United States has many more machines per capita, the staffing per machine is much less favorable, perhaps because many of our machines are not used heavily. Letter from Dr. James J. Diamond, October 21, 1981.

31. According to R. C. Lawson, chairman of the professional committee of the Hospital Physicists Association in London, there were 110 to 115 physicists in radiotherapy in Britain in 1981. The Hospital Physicists Association also estimates that one physicist is required per 500 new patients a year, or about 190 physicists. By this criterion the United States would need about 700 physicists. The actual number lies between 700 and 1,000. In November 1981 Dr. Bengt Bjarngard of the Department of Radiation Therapy, Massachusetts General Hospital, estimated that there were about 700 qualified full-time-equivalent physicists in radiotherapy. The estimate was based on an analysis of the membership in 1980 of the American Association of Physicists in Medicine with methods reported by the Committee for Radiology Oncology Studies, "Research Plan for Radiation Oncology," *Cancer,* vol. 37 (April supplement, 1976), pp. 2040–148. In a letter, October 21, 1981, Dr. James J. Diamond reported that a survey of 90 percent of U.S. radiotherapy facilities had revealed 643 full-time and 671 part-time physicists. Weighting part-time physicists as one-third of full-time yields an estimate of 867 full-time equivalents. If the other 10 percent of facilities were identically staffed, the total number would be 963. The difference between that figure and Bjarngard's lower one probably lies in Bjarngard's reference to "qualified" physicists.

32. Vincent T. DeVita, Jr., "Principles of Cancer Therapy," in Kurt J. Isselbacher and others, eds., *Harrison's Principles of Internal Medicine,* 9th ed. (McGraw-Hill, 1980). pp. 1597–1620.

33. Letter from Dr. George Canellos, chief of the division of medical oncology, Sidney Farber Cancer Institute, August 11, 1982. These estimates take into account that not all patients receive treatment for a full year. Some die and some drop out. The estimates assume an average of eight months of treatment per patient.

34. Data from IMS America, Ltd., provided by James Donahue, April 13, 1982; and letter from Dr. Arthur S. Levine, assistant director for science, National Cancer Institute, August 11, 1982.

35. Letters from Dr. Arthur S. Levine, August 11, 1982, and from American Society of Clinical Oncology, August 11, 1982. More than 1,600 oncologists are board-certified. They are widely diffused geographically. Relatively small communities, such as Pocatello, Idaho; Gallipolis, Ohio; and Wood, Wisconsin, now have at least one such certified oncologist. See *Marquis Directory of Medical Specialists, 1981–1982,* pp. 1343–49.

36. Data from IMS America, Ltd., provided by James Donahue.

37. Testicular tumors, choriocarcinoma, and other curable cancers are usually referred to specialized centers and receive the best treatment modern medicine has to offer. Treatment of patients with Hodgkin's disease is often carried out in peripheral hospitals. Although the British consider the management of such cases to be part of basic medical knowledge, care in those hospitals is probably not as good as it would be in specialized centers.

38. Information on adjuvant therapy was provided in letters from Dr. T. J. McElwain, Royal Marsden Hospital, London, August 2, 1982; Dr. Ray Powles, August 4, 1982; and Dr. Derek Crowther, head of Department of Medical Oncology, University of Manchester, August 26, 1982. Information on drug regimens in Britain was provided in letters from Professor K. D. Bagshawe, Charing Cross Hospital Medical School, May 26, 1982, and Dr. T. J. McElwain, June 16, 1982. Data on sales of cancer chemotherapeutic agents came from James Donahue. Dr. Steven W. Papish, Hematology-Oncology Service, Tufts–New England Medical Center, analyzed these data.

39. J. V. Watson, "What Does 'Response' in Cancer Chemotherapy Really Mean?" *British Medical Journal,* vol. 283 (July 1981), pp. 34–37.

40. C. G. Moertel, "ASCO (American Society of Clinical Oncology) Presidential Address, 1980," *Medical and Pediatric Oncology,* vol. 8, no. 3 (1980), pp. 215–20.

41. Letter to the authors from Dr. R. J. Wrighton, Department of Health and Social Security, July 2, 1982.

42. A minority of cases of aplastic anemia are caused by specific drugs and toxins, but in approximately 50 to 70 percent of cases the etiology is unknown. J. M. Rappeport and H. Franklin Bunn, "Bone Marrow Failure: Aplastic Anemia and Other Disorders of the Bone Marrow," in Isselbacher and others, eds., *Harrison's Principles of Internal Medicine,* pp. 1525–30; Robert Peter Gale, "Aplastic Anemia: Biology and Treatment," *Annals of Internal Medicine,* vol. 95 (October 1981), pp. 477–94; and Mortimer M. Bortin and others, "Allogenic Bone Marrow Transplantation for 144 Patients with Severe Aplastic Anemia," *Journal of the American Medical Association,* vol. 245 (March 20, 1981), pp. 1132–39.

43. The two groups of leukemics for whom the outlook is grim with continued chemotherapy but seems to be better with BMT are (1) patients with acute lymphocytic leukemia who have twice enjoyed periods of remission after treatment but have relapsed again; and (2) those with acute myelogenous leukemia in first remission. E. Donnall Thomas, "Bone Marrow Transplantation: Present Status and Future Expectations," in Isselbacher and others, eds., *Harrison's Principles of Internal Medicine, Update I* (McGraw-Hill, 1980), pp. 135–52.

44. Bortin and others, "Allogenic Bone Marrow Transplantation."

45. E. Donnall Thomas, "The Role of Marrow Transplantation in the Eradication of Malignant Disease," *Cancer,* vol. 49 (May 15, 1982), pp. 1963–69; and Robert Peter Gale, "Progress in Bone Marrow Transplantation in Man," *Survey of Immunologic Research,* vol. 1 (1982), pp. 40-66.

46. Letters from Dr. E. Donnall Thomas, Division of Oncology, Department of Medicine, University of Washington, August 26, 1982, and Dr. Robert Peter Gale, UCLA School of Medicine, August 27, 1982; and R. J. Wrighton, "Bone Marrow Transplantation (BMT)" (DHSS, 1982). The data presented here were obtained from the Statistical Center of the International Bone Marrow Transplant Registry. The analysis has not been reviewed or approved by the advisory committee of the registry.

47. U.S. costs are from S. O. Schweitzer and C. C. Scalzi, *The Cost-Effectiveness of Bone Marrow Transplant Therapy and Its Policy Implications: The Implications of Cost-Effectiveness of Medical Technology* (U.S. Office of Technology Assessment, 1981); and letter from Dr. E. Donnall Thomas, August 26, 1982. British costs are from

Wrighton, "Bone Marrow Transplantation"; J. R. Hobbs, "Bone Marrow Transplantation for Inborn Errors," *Lancet,* vol. 2 (October 3, 1981), pp. 735–39; and H. E. M. Kay and others, "Cost of Bone-Marrow Transplants in Acute Myeloid Leukemia," *Lancet,* vol. 1 (May 17, 1980), pp. 1067–69. The figures quoted by these authors do not include any allowance for interest or depreciation and so are probably several thousand dollars too low.

48. J. E. Fischer, "Hyperalimentation," in Charles Rob, ed., *Advances in Surgery,* vol. 11 (Chicago: Year Book Publishers, 1977), pp. 1–69.

49. On the value of TPN, see J. T. Goodgame, Jr., "A Critical Assessment of the Indications for Total Parenteral Nutrition," *Surgery, Gynecology, and Obstetrics,* vol. 151 (1980), pp. 433–41; J. M. Muller and others, "Preoperative Parenteral Feeding in Patients with Gastrointestinal Carcinoma," *Lancet,* vol. 1 (1982), pp. 66–71; J. L. Mullen and others, "Reduction of Operative Morbidity and Mortality by Combined Preoperative and Postoperative Nutritional Support," *Annals of Surgery,* vol. 192 (1980), pp. 604–13; M. F. Brennan, "Total Parenteral Nutrition in the Cancer Patient," *New England Journal of Medicine,* vol. 305 (August 13, 1981), pp. 375–82; E. M. Copeland, "Total Parenteral Nutrition in Cancer," *New England Journal of Medicine,* vol. 305 (December 1981), pp. 1589–90; and Fischer, "Hyperalimentation."

50. F. T. Padberg and others, "Central Venous Catheterization for Parenteral Nutrition," *Annals of Surgery,* vol. 193 (1981), pp. 264–70.

51. For hospital costs, see L. P. Wateska and others, "Cost of a Home Parenteral Nutrition Program," *Journal of the American Medical Association,* vol. 244 (November 1980), pp. 2303–04; W. J. Byrne and others, "Home Parenteral Nutrition," *Surgery, Gynecology, and Obstetrics,* vol. 149 (October 1979), pp. 593–99; and Goodgame, "Critical Assessment." Goodgame's figure of $250 to $300 a day specifically excludes the cost of the hospital room and standard nursing care, whereas Wateska and others' figure of $200 a day includes the cost of hospitalization. (Letter from Leon P. Wateska, director of hospital pharmacy, Cleveland Clinic, Cleveland, Ohio.) For home costs, see Fischer, "Hyperalimentation"; Wateska and others, "Cost of a Home Parenteral Nutrition Program"; C. R. Fleming and others, "Home Parenteral Nutrition for Management of the Severely Malnourished Adult Patient," *Gastroenterology,* vol. 79 (July 1980), pp. 11–18; Byrne and others, "Home Parenteral Nutrition"; and C. D. Lees and others, "Home Parenteral Nutrition," *Surgical Clinics of North America,* vol. 61 (1981), pp. 621–22.

52. This estimate is based on a conversion factor of two dollars to a pound. M. Irving, "Home Parenteral Nutrition in the United Kingdom," 2d European Congress on Parenteral and Enteral Nutrition, Newcastle upon Tyne, September 7–10, 1980; *Acta Chirurgica Scandinavica,* supplement 507 (1981), pp. 140–42; and P. J. Milewski and others, "Parenteral Nutrition at Home in Management of Intestinal Failure," *British Medical Journal,* vol. 280 (June 1980), pp. 1356–57.

53. Letter from Donald R. Kiepert, Jr., Travenol Laboratories, October 21, 1980. Because the cost per unit of amino acid was slightly higher in Britain than in the United States, the number of units used per capita was less than one-fifth of the number used in the United States.

54. Memorandum from Joseph M. Sceppa, associate director of administrative services, Department of Pharmacy, New England Medical Center, December 12, 1980. The calculation of total expenditures is based on the finding that about half the cost of TPN administration was attributable to factors other than the solution itself—nursing services, tubing, laboratory tests, and so on.

55. Schwartz and Joskow, "Duplicated Hospital Facilities," pp. 1449–57; and HCFA, *End-Stage Renal Disease,* p. 1.

**Chapter 4 (pages 57–67)**

1. Philip Wood, ed., *Challenge of Arthritis and Rheumatism: A Report on Problems and Progress in Health Care for Rheumatic Disorders* (London: Her Majesty's Stationery Office, 1977), p. 48; and *Orthopaedic Services: Waiting Time for Out-Patient Appointments and In-Patient Treatment,* Report of Working Party to the Secretary of State for Social Services (HMSO, 1981), p. 4.

2. R. B. Buttery and others, "Surgical Provision, Waiting Times, and Waiting Lists," *Health Trends,* vol. 12 (August 1980), pp. 57–61.

3. J. Charnley, the discoverer of polymethylmethacrylate, reports that well under 1 percent a year of the hips he has replaced require surgery because of loosening. See A. J. Harrold, "Outlook for Hip Replacement," *British Medical Journal,* vol. 284 (January 16, 1982), p. 139. This article also reports a failure rate of 54 percent over five years for patients under thirty.

4. The waiting time of patients before treatment could average as little as one year or be much longer. Given a waiting list equal to the number of patients treated in one year, there would be a one-year average waiting time if patients were admitted on a first-come, first-served basis. If the severest cases were admitted first, there would be a longer average waiting time; in that event, the waiting list would largely consist of those who had problems not severe enough to merit treatment and who might remain on the list for many years. In fact, 80 percent of all hospital admissions in Britain occur without delay, suggesting that the second model is closer to reality than the first. See Jeremy Hurst, "Financing Health Services in the United States, Canada, and Britain," Nuffield/Levesholme Fellowship Report (November 1982), p. 90.

5. This is a rough estimate, based on the report that in 1975 there were 12,000 patients awaiting hip arthroplasty (total joint replacement), according to J. R. Morris, "Analysis of Services Available for Total Joint Replacement Surgery," *British Medical Journal,* vol. 3 (August 1975), p. 290; and the report that in 1972 and 1977, respectively, 18,980 and 27,080 hip arthroplasties were performed in England and Wales, in *Orthopaedic Services,* p. 20.

6. W. J. Modle, "Trends and Problems" (Department of Health and Social Security, 1979), p. 4; *Orthopaedic Services,* pp. 10–11.

7. *Orthopaedic Services,* pp. 16, 21.

8. Ibid., p. 43; Modle, "Trends and Problems," p. 5; and interviews.

9. Interviews with the authors.

10. Harold S. Luft and others, "Should Operations Be Regionalized? The Empirical Relation Between Surgical Volume and Mortality," *New England Journal of Medicine,* vol. 301 (December 20, 1979), p. 1365.

11. "Special Report," National Center for Health Care Technology, Technology Assessment Forum, Coronary Artery Bypass Surgery, June 23, 1981, pp. 1, 4, 8; "Coronary Artery Bypass Surgery—Indications and Limitations," *Lancet,* vol. 2 (September 6, 1980), p. 511; and Gina Kolata, "Some Bypass Surgery Unnecessary," *Science,* vol. 222 (November 11, 1983), p. 605.

12. National Institutes of Health Consensus Development Conference, "Coronary Artery Bypass Surgery: Scientific and Clinical Aspects," *New England Journal of Medicine,* vol. 304 (March 12, 1981), pp. 680–84. According to a U.S. Veterans Administration study, the four-year survival rates for patients with severe left main artery disease were 89 percent for surgically treated patients and 60 percent for medically treated ones. According to a European randomized study, the comparable survival rates for three vessel disease were 89 percent and 67 percent.

13. The British estimate is from Kolata, "Consensus on Bypass Surgery," p. 42. U.S. estimates are from Office of Technology Assessment, *The Implications of Cost Effectiveness Analysis of Medical Technology,* Background Paper 4: *The Management of Health Care Technology in Ten Countries* (Washington, D.C.: OTA, 1980), p. 212. Other sources are qualitatively consistent with this estimate, though the precise numbers differ. In 1976, 21,290 heart operations of all kinds were performed in England and Wales, but of these only 880 were for "operations affecting myocardium," 320 for "combined open heart operations," and 310 for "grafts for repair of vessel." (Letter from P. W. Annesley of DHSS, August 1979.) The rest were pacemaker insertions, catheter manipulations, or work on valves or the septum within the heart cavity. According to Dr. Prophet of DHSS, in the United Kingdom the rate per million of all "open heart surgery" was 178 per million in 1978 (compared with 800 per million in Australia); of this total 59 were for IHD (presumably ischemic heart disease) and include all coronary artery bypass cases. That implies roughly 3,400 operations. Another source reports 55 coronary artery bypasses per million population in England and Wales in 1978. This nationwide average in Britain conceals large differences across the nation; the rate in 1978 was 120 per million in the four Thames regions and averaged about 35 elsewhere. Of the 120, 30 were referred from other regions.

14. Richard Cooper, "Rising Death Rates in the Soviet Union—The Impact of Coronary Heart Disease," *New England Journal of Medicine,* vol. 304 (May 21, 1981), p. 1262.

15. Matt Clark, "A Whole New Class of Heart Drugs," *Newsweek,* March 30, 1981; "Nifedipine (Adalat) for Angina," *Drug and Therapeutics Bulletin,* vol. 17 (March 1979), pp. 22–24; A. C. F. Kenmore and J. H. Scrutton, "A Double-Blind Controlled Trial of the Anti-Anginal Efficacy of Nifedipine Compared with Propranolol," *British Journal of Clinical Practice,* vol. 33 (February 1979), p. 49; John Raftos, "Verapamil in the Long-Term Treatment of Angina Pectoris," *Medical Journal of Australia,* vol. 2 (July 1980), p. 78; C. de Ponti and others, "Comparative Effects of Nifedipine, Verapamil, Isosorbide Dinitrate and Propranolol on Exercise-Induced Angina Pectoris," *European Journal of Cardiology,* vol. 10 (January 1979), p. 47; Elliott Antman and others, "Nifedipine Therapy for Coronary-Artery Spasm," *New England Journal of Medicine,* vol. 302 (June 5, 1980), p. 1269; and Peter Lynch and others, "Objective Assessment of Antianginal Treatment: A Double-Blind Comparison of Propranolol, Nifedipine and Their Combination," *British Medical Journal,* vol. 281 (July 1980), p. 184.

16. This statement is based on the assumption that 40 percent of angiographic studies indicate three vessel or left main artery disease in Britain as in the United States, and that the frequency of indications for surgery is proportional to age-adjusted death rates from coronary disease reported above. By ignoring the recent U.S. decline in deaths from coronary disease and the greater proportion of elderly in Britain than in the United States, the text estimate understates the relative number of cases in which surgery is indicated in Britain. The most recent results from a sample of European patients with coronary heart disease show that surgery may improve life expectancy in many other cases as well. "Long-Term Results of Prospective Randomised Study of Coronary Artery Bypass Surgery in Stable Angina Pectoris," *Lancet,* vol. 2 (November 27, 1982), pp. 1173–80.

17. "Coronary Artery Bypass Surgery—Indications and Limitations," p. 512.

18. NIH Consensus Development Conference, "Coronary Artery Bypass Surgery."

19. Kolata, "Consensus on Bypass Surgery," p. 43.

20. John P. Bunker, M.D., "Surgical Manpower: A Comparison of Operations and Surgeons in the United States and in England and Wales," *New England Journal of Medicine,* vol. 282 (January 15, 1970), pp. 135–44.

Chapter 5 (pages 68–76)

1. William Schwartz, "Decision Analysis: A Look at the Chief Complaints," *New England Journal of Medicine,* vol. 300 (March 8, 1979), pp. 556–60.

2. Office of Technology Assessment, *Policy Implications of the Computed Tomography (CT) Scanner: An Update* (Washington, D.C.: OTA, 1981), pp. 59–71; National Institutes of Health, "Computed Tomographic Scanning of the Brain," Consensus Development Conference statement, November 4–6, 1981. These procedures include the dynamic spatial reconstructor, which will allow "accurate imaging of moving organ systems"; positron emission transaxial tomography and single photon emission computed tomography, in which radioactive isotopes are injected and traced; zeugmatography, a means of creating a two- or three-dimensional image using nuclear magnetic resonance, a technique using nonionizing forms of energy to produce sectional images of the human body. Recent improvements in ultrasound instrumentation have allowed far more sophisticated use of ultrasonography. For a fairly nontechnical explanation of nuclear magnetic resonance and its applications, see R. G. Shulman, "NMR Spectroscopy of Living Cells," *Scientific American,* vol. 248 (January 1983), pp. 86–93.

3. Gina Kolata, "Consensus on CT Scans," *Science,* vol. 214 (December 18, 1981), pp. 1327–28; and National Institutes of Health, "Computer Tomographic Scanning of the Brain," p. 2.

4. OTA, *Policy Implications of the CT Scanner,* pp. 23, 60; Ronald G. Evens and R. Gilbert Jost, "Economic Analysis of Body Computed Tomography Units Including Data on Utilization," *Radiology,* vol. 127 (April 1978), pp. 151–56; and William B. Schwartz and Paul L. Joskow, "Duplicated Hospital Facilities: How Much Can We Save by Consolidating Them?" *New England Journal of Medicine,* vol. 303 (December 18, 1980), pp. 1449–57.

5. The $25 estimate of marginal cost is based on Evens and Jost, "Economic Analysis of Body Computed Tomography Units," p. 156.

6. Ibid.; and G. M. K. Hughes, "National Survey of Computed Tomography Unit Capacity," *Radiology,* vol. 135 (June 1980), p. 701. The resource cost per scan varies markedly by type of scan. Head scans without contrast media require 33 minutes; body studies with contrast media require 56 minutes; dual studies (scans both with and without contrast media) average 58 minutes for head studies and 83 minutes for body studies. Variations from one facility to another within types of studies are even larger. On congested units time is a good measure of relative average cost; on uncongested units time is a good measure of relative marginal cost.

7. Compare Department of Health and Social Security, "Whole Body CT Scanners in England and Wales" (DHSS, 1980), with Evens and Jost, "Economic Analysis of Body Computed Tomography Units."

8. According to the Office of Technology Assessment, the United States had 400 head scanners and 854 body scanners in 1979 and 460 head scanners and 1,011 body scanners in 1980. See OTA, *Policy Implications of the CT Scanner,* pp. 15–17. An additional 395 to 435 scanners were shipped in 1981. "Market Scan: CT Scanning Redux," *Diagnostic Imaging* (April 1982), p. 15. In 1979 the United Kingdom had 39 head scanners and 18 body scanners. In 1980 England and Wales had 21 body scanners installed and 12 on order. DHSS, "Whole Body CT Scanners in England and Wales," p. 1. Per million population, the United States had 1.78 head scanners and 3.80 body scanners in 1979, and 2.03 head scanners and 4.45 body scanners in 1980. The United Kingdom had 0.69 head scanners and 0.32 body scanners per million population in 1979, and England and Wales had 0.43 body scanners per million population installed in 1980.

9. Kolata, "Consensus on CT Scans," pp. 1327–28.

10. The United States did a weekly average of 34 scans per body scanner and 63 scans per head scanner in 1979, according to Ronald G. Evens and R. Gilbert Jost, "Utilization of Head Computed Tomography Units," *Radiology*, vol. 131 (June 1979), p. 691, and "Utilization of Body Computed Tomography Units," ibid., p. 696. These averages translate into a total of 1,787,448 scans on body scanners and 1,506,960 scans on head scanners annually, a rate of 7,767 scans per million population on body scanners, 6,633 per million on head scanners, and 14,500 per million overall. Fifty-five percent of all scans done on body scanners are done on heads. The Office of Technology Assessment estimates that 3 to 4 million CT scans of all kinds were done in the United States in 1980. See OTA, *Policy Implications of the CT Scanner*, p. 59. Evens and Jost take their estimates from centers where body scanners have been in operation at least eighteen months and head scanners have been in operation at least thirty months. Because new centers do fewer procedures than experienced ones, Evens and Jost's estimates may be too high for the average U.S. facility.

For Britain, the data are less good. DHSS reports in "Whole Body CT Scanners in England and Wales," p. 9, that five centers with body scanners did an average of 1,817 scans in 1979. An EMI brain scanner at the Frenchay Hospital was used for 4,012 patients in the second year of operation, up from 2,012 during the first year, according to J. L. G. Thomson, "Cost Effectiveness of an EMI Brain Scanner: A Review of a 2-Year Experience," *Health Trends*, vol. 9 (February 1977), p. 18. A target of at least 2,750 scans a year was suggested by J. R. Bartlett and others, "Evaluating Cost Effectiveness of Diagnostic Equipment: The Brain Scanner Case," *British Medical Journal*, vol. 2 (September 16, 1978), p. 817. F. G. M. Ross, "Report of Royal College of Radiologists: Members of the Working Party on CT Scanning" (London, November 12, 1979), p. 6, stated that "the throughput of patients per day varies greatly with the purpose for which the scanner is being used (brain approximately 15–18 per working day, body approximately 8–10 per working day)." It is not clear whether this statement refers to actual or ideal practice.

11. DHSS, "Whole Body Scanners in England and Wales, p. 1.

12. See data from G. M. Kendall and others, "A Frequency Survey of Radiological Examinations Carried Out in National Health Service Hospitals in Great Britain in 1977 for Diagnostic Purposes," National Radiological Protection Board (HMSO, June 1980); Bureau of Radiological Health, "Cost Containment Planning Document" (August 1978), app. 4, p. 72; and Bruce Hillman and others, "Simplifying Radiological Examinations— the Urogram as a Model," *Lancet*, vol. 1 (May 19, 1979), pp. 1068–71. In 1977 Britain performed 438 medical and 212 dental diagnostic x-rays per thousand population through the NHS and private medicine. The United States performed 728 medical and 387 dental x-rays per thousand population. Separate estimates by Eastman Kodak put the total number of x-rays in 1980 at 1,277 per thousand population.

The NHS hospitals used 55 million square feet of x-ray film in 1977 and 59 million square feet in 1978; the United States used 846 and 896 million square feet, respectively. See Dr. Ronald Oliver, "Consumption of Radiographic Film in NHS Hospitals, Great Britain" and *Wolfman Report on the Photographic Industry in the U.S.* (Modern Photography Magazine, 1979–80). The United States used 3.89 times as much x-ray film per capita in 1977 as did Great Britain, and 3.80 times as much in 1978.

13. R. J. Wrighton and R. M. Oliver, "Trends in Radiological Practice in the NHS," *Health Trends*, vol. 12 (May 1980), p. 22.

14. American Medical Association, *Profiles of Medical Practice 1980* (AMA, 1980), p. 145; and Wrighton and Oliver, "Trends in Radiological Practice," p. 22.

15. According to Charles R. Pross, an executive with the National Electrical

Manufacturers Association, the United States spent $714 million on medical diagnostic x-ray equipment in 1979, excluding CT scanners, dental x-rays, and industrial x-ray and radiotherapy equipment. According to A. Burchell, a DHSS official, the NHS spent $43 million (converted from pounds to dollars by the average IMF exchange rates published in *International Financial Statistics*) in the same year. These figures translate into $3.24 per capita in the United States and $0.88 per capita in England and Wales.

16. For the British estimate, see Wrighton and Oliver, "Trends in Radiological Practice," and letter from A. Burchell, September 5, 1980; for the U.S. figures, see Bureau of Radiological Health, "Cost Containment Planning Document," app. 4.

17. The danger of such excessive examination is exacerbated by the fact that many machines are poorly calibrated and deliver dosages far greater than the minimum necessary to produce a reliable picture. U.S. Food and Drug Administration, "A Proposed FDA Program to Reduce Unnecessary Patient Exposure from Diagnostic X-rays: Cost Containment Considerations," working paper (August 1978), app. 3.


**Chapter 6 (pages 79–88)**

1. Joseph P. Newhouse, "Medical Care Expenditure: A Cross-National Survey," *Journal of Human Resources*, vol. 12 (Winter, 1977), pp. 115–25; and J. R. Richardson, "The Costs and Benefits of Health Care Services: Some International Evidence," in R. Mendelsohn, ed., *Social Welfare Finance: Selected Papers* (Australian National University, 1982), pp. 139–54.

2. Alan Williams, "Efficiency and Welfare," in Sir Douglas Black and G. P. Thomas, eds., *Providing for the Health Services* (London: Croom Helm, 1978), pp. 31–32.

3. Richard Cooper, "Rising Death Rates in the Soviet Union," *New England Journal of Medicine*, vol. 304 (May 21, 1981), p. 1262; Department of Health and Social Security, *Health and Personal Social Services Statistics for England, 1982* (London: Her Majesty's Stationery Office, 1982), p. 13; and U.S. Department of Commerce, *Preliminary Estimates of the Population of the United States, by Age, Sex, and Race, 1970 to 1981*, Population Estimates and Projections, series P-25, no. 917 (Government Printing Office, 1982), pp. 9–10. In 1978 the per capita health expenditure in Great Britain for prime-age adults (aged sixteen through sixty-four) was £85, a far smaller amount than the £400 spent on those over sixty-five. Similarly, in the United States the per capita expenditure for prime-age adults (aged nineteen through sixty-four) was $764, compared with $2,026 spent on those over sixty-five. *The Government's Expenditure Plans, 1980–81 to 1983–84* (HMSO, 1980), p. 104; and Charles R. Fisher, "Differences by Age Groups in Health Care Spending," *Health Care Financing Review*, vol. 1 (Spring 1980), p. 66.

4. In 1960 the United States spent $149.28 per capita on all health services and the British spent $46.03 (at the exchange rate for that year of $2.80 = £1). In 1978 prices, based on the U.S. GNP deflator, the expenditures were $326.04 in the United States and $100.54 in Britain. Assuming that the adjustments we made in table 6-1 would have reduced spending by the same fraction in 1960 as they did in 1978, these numbers become $123.73 for the United States and $56.71 for Britain, a difference of $67.02.


**Chapter 7 (pages 89–112)**

1. To arrive at this figure, we calculated the number of people on dialysis per million in the United States. We multiplied this rate by the British population (in millions) and the British costs, then divided that number by British health expenditures.

2. Gywn Bevan and others, *Health Care Priorities and Management* (London: Croom Helm, 1980), p. 169; and Department of Health and Social Security, *Health and Personal Social Services Statistics for England, 1978* (Her Majesty's Stationery Office, 1978), p. 29. A kidney failure rate of 190 per million (a high estimate) would lead to an average annual rate of 0.4 cases per general practitioner.

3. Authors' estimate based on inspection of unpublished statistical reports of the Department of Health and Social Security (SH3 Reports, various years). Our direct observations seem consistent with this estimate. The range of the estimate is broad because there does not appear to be any standard definition of "intensive care beds" and reporting is spotty.

4. For British data, see *The Government's Expenditure Plans, 1980–81 to 1983–84* (HMSO, 1980), p. 104. For U.S. data, see Charles R. Fisher, "Differences by Age Groups in Health Care Spending," *Health Care Financing Review*, vol. 1 (Spring 1980), p. 81. Because the programs covered in the two sources are so different, the numbers in the text are approximations.

5. Figures are inflation-adjusted five-year averages. For the British figure, see Central Statistical Office, *National Income and Expenditure* (HMSO, 1979), p. 80. For the U.S. figure, see U.S. Department of Commerce, *Statistical Abstract of the United States, 1981* (Government Printing Office, 1981), p. 751.

6. Rodney Deitch, "A Cash Limit on Family Practitioner Services?" *Lancet*, vol. 2 (August 8, 1981), pp. 317–18. Subsequently the Greenfield report rejected the idea of limiting free prescriptions by GPs to a formulary of approved drugs. See "Effective Prescribing," *British Medical Journal*, vol. 286 (February 12, 1983), p. 567.

7. Robin Dowie, "National Trends in Domiciliary Consultations," *British Medical Journal*, vol. 286 (March 5, 1983), pp. 819–22. Part of the increase occurred because the British population has been aging and the rate of home visits by consultants in geriatric medicine and mental illness is higher than for other specialists.

8. *Royal Commission on the National Health Service Report* (HMSO, 1979), p. 289.

9. Office of Health Economics, *Hip Replacement and the NHS* (London: White Crescent Press, 1982).

10. Department of Health, Education, and Welfare, "The Malpractice Problem in Great Britain," appendix to *Report of the Secretary's Commission on Medical Malpractice, 1973* (GPO, 1973); and correspondence with J. W. Brooke Barnett, secretary of the Medical Defence Union, April 11, 1983.

11. *Medical Defence Union Annual Report, 1982;* and HEW, "Malpractice Problem in Great Britain."

12. Office of Health Economics, *Renal Failure: A Priority in Health?* (London: White Crescent Press, 1978).

13. R. J. Wrighton, "Bone Marrow Transplantation" (DHSS, 1982).

14. Rodney Deitch, "Bone Marrow Transplants: Commentary from Westminster," *Lancet*, vol. 2 (December 12, 1981), p. 1355.

**Chapter 8 (pages 113–35)**

1. Robert J. Myers, "Financial Status of the Social Security Program," *Social Security Bulletin*, vol. 46 (March 1983), p. 13.

2. Liz Roman Gallese, "Massachusetts Law Offers New Approach to Cut Hospital Costs," *Wall Street Journal*, August 13, 1982; Jean Dietz, "Hospital Chiefs Draft Cuts under New Cost Control Law," *Boston Globe*, September 30, 1982; and Edward Melia

and others, "Competition in the Health Care Market-Place: A Beginning in California," *New England Journal of Medicine,* vol. 308 (March 31, 1983), pp. 788–92.

3. For an examination of these issues, see Stephen Breyer, *Regulation and Its Reform* (Harvard University Press, 1982).

4. William B. Schwartz and Paul L. Joskow, "Duplicated Hospital Facilities: How Much Can We Save by Consolidating Them?" *New England Journal of Medicine,* vol. 303 (December 18, 1980), pp. 1449–57.

5. Ibid.

6. Aviva A. Berk and Thomas C. Chalmers, "Cost and Efficacy of the Substitution of Ambulatory for Inpatient Care," *New England Journal of Medicine,* vol. 304 (February 12, 1981), pp. 393–97; and Richard A. Elnicki, "Substitution of Outpatient for Inpatient Hospital Care: A Cost Analysis," *Inquiry,* vol. 13 (September 1976), pp. 245–61.

7. American Hospital Association, *Hospital Statistics, 1981* (Chicago: AHA, 1981). Outpatient visits rose 7.2 percent a year from 1965 through 1976 but declined slightly in the next four years.

8. William B. Schwartz and Paul L. Joskow, "Medical Efficacy versus Economic Efficiency: A Conflict in Values," *New England Journal of Medicine,* vol. 299 (December 28, 1978), pp. 1462–64.

9. Ibid.

10. Harold S. Luft, *Health Maintenance Organizations: Dimensions of Performance* (Wiley, 1981), pp. 60–61. These estimates must be viewed cautiously because they are based on a small number of studies and do not adjust for differences in the populations that join the various plans.

11. The unlimited exclusion of employer-financed health benefits from the employee's income means that the employee cannot "take out in wages" the savings from health maintenance organizations without paying tax on such increased wages; the employer, likewise, would reap only part of the savings, because a reduction of labor costs, other things equal, increases taxable profits, causing savings on health insurance to increase his taxes.

12. As of January 1978, the rate-setting bureau faced a backlog of 2,400 suits. Diane Hamilton and Gilby Kamens, "Prospective Reimbursement in New York," *Topics in Health Care Financing,* vol. 6 (1979), pp. 97–108.

13. William B. Schwartz, "The Regulation Strategy for Controlling Hospital Costs: Problems and Prospects," *New England Journal of Medicine,* vol. 305 (November 19, 1981), pp. 1249–55.

14. R. Alsop, "U.S. Efforts to Control Hospital Growth Costs Meet Wide Opposition," *Wall Street Journal,* March 20, 1978; T. Chamberlain, "Small Towns Mobilize to Save Their Hospitals," *Boston Globe,* January 31, 1979; E. Hudson, "Opposition Is Heated to a Decrease in Maternity Wards in 7 Counties," *New York Times,* June 17, 1977; and H. Nelson, "Cutting Hospital Costs No Easy Task," *Los Angeles Times,* July 20, 1977.

15. See John P. Bunker, "Surgical Manpower: A Comparison of Operations and Surgeons in the United States and in England and Wales," *New England Journal of Medicine,* vol. 302 (January 15, 1980), pp. 135–44.

16. A recent analysis suggests that the choice would make little medical difference: W. B. Schwartz and P. L. Joskow, Memorandum, Boston, 1980.

17. Erich H. Loewy, "Cost Should Not Be a Factor in Medical Care," *New England Journal of Medicine,* vol. 302 (March 20, 1980), p. 697.

18. This problem, known as moral hazard, is common to many forms of insurance. For example, burglary insurance reduces the incentive of homeowners to buy pickproof locks, alarm systems, or other devices to discourage burglars.

19. William B. Schwartz and Neil K. Komesar, "Doctors, Damages and Deterrence: An Economic View of Medical Malpractice," *New England Journal of Medicine,* vol. 298 (June 8, 1978), pp. 1282–89.

## Appendix (pages 137–38)

1. Joseph Melton, III, M.D., and others, "Rates of Total Hip Arthroplasty: A Population Based Study," *New England Journal of Medicine,* vol. 307 (November 11, 1982), p. 1242. A similar estimate is reported in "Total Hip-Joint Replacement in the United States," *Journal of the American Medical Association,* vol. 248 (October 15, 1982), pp. 1817–21. This source reports that 75,000 total hip replacements were performed on 65,000 patients in an unstated annual period in the United States.

# Index

Aged: British hospital care, 86n; hip replacement surgery, 59; medical resource allocation for, 8, 36–37, 90, 97, 104, 110
Angina pectoris, 57; bypass surgery for, 28, 56, 62–64; described, 62; drug therapy for, 64–65, 93

Bevan, Aneurin, 21–22
Bone marrow transplantation (BMT), 28, 75; British resource allocation for, 94; cost, 52; described, 50–51; as political issue, 109–10; risk, 51–52
British Renal Association, 109
Budget. *See* Medical budget

California, medicaid costs control program, 115
Cancer, 8, 28; chemotherapy, 44–50, 93–94; radiotherapy, 40–44, 93
Carter, Jimmy, 4, 116
Certificate of need (CON) programs, 5
Charitable donations of medical equipment, 10; CT scanners, 71, 95, 105–06; in response to budget limits, 20, 130–31; tax deductibility, 105
Chemotherapy, 28, 74; Britain, 47–50; cost, 46, 48; drugs, 45; resource allocation for, 93–94; United States, 46–47, 48–49; use, 44–46
Clinical freedom, 9–10, 102–04
Computed tomographic (CT) scanners, 28, 56, 75; capacity for, 71; charitable donations of, 71, 95, 105–06; cost, 70–71, 83n; described, 69; future use, 72; resource allocation for, 94–95
CON programs. *See* Certificate of need programs
Consultants, British, 10; NHS, 15, 16; private practice, 22
Coronary artery surgery, 28, 56, 62, 74, 75; attitudes toward, 65–67; cost, 63,

67; described, 62–63; resource allocation for, 92–93
Costs, medical: benefits versus, 81, 83, 98; bone marrow transplantation, 52; chemotherapy, 46, 48; coronary artery surgery, 63, 67; CT scans, 70–71; dialysis, 32, 35, 118; hemophilia treatment, 39; new technology, 125–26; radiotherapy, 44; total parenteral nutrition, 54–55
CT scanners. *See* Computed tomographic scanners

Diagnostic related groupings (DRG), 114, 119–20
Diagnostic techniques, 68–69. *See also* Computed tomographic scanners; X-ray services
Dialysis, 28; British resource constraints on, 34–37; cost, 32, 33, 35, 118; effects, 31; hemodialysis, 29–30; home program, 33–34; peritoneal, 30; rates of treatment, 32–33, 34n
DRG. *See* Diagnostic related groupings
Drugs: heart disease, 64–65; international price differences for, 86n; NHS provisions for, 17

Efficiency, medical: benefits from, 80–83; explained, 79, 89
Equipment, medical, 8; British-U.S. expenditures on, 87–88; budget limits and, 19, 41–42; charitable gifts of, 10, 20, 71, 130–31; international price differences for, 86n
Expenditures. *See* Hospital expenditures; Medical expenditures

Ford, Gerald M., 4, 116

Health and Human Services, Department of (HHS), 5, 116

159